MASSAGE NATIONAL EXAM
Questions and Answers

**Daphna R. Moore, CMT, NA and Massage Instructor
in Denver and Boulder, Colorado**
Retired Member of AMTA

Hughes Henshaw Publications
Denver, CO 80226-1642

Library of Congress in Catalog Publication Data

**MOORE, DAPHNA CMT, RETIRED MEMBER OF AMTA
MASSAGE INSTRUCTOR COLORADO AND GINA PERRUSQUIA**

MASSAGE NATIONAL EXAM QUESTIONS AND ANSWERS

ISBN 1-892693-08-9
Copyright © 1993, 1994, 1995, 1997, 1999, and 2000 by Daphna R. Moore
First Printing 1993
Second Printing 1994, revised
Third Printing 1995, revised
Fourth Printing 1997
Fifth Printing 1999
Sixth Printing 2000 completely revised

Printed in the United States of America

**INTERNATIONAL STANDARD BOOK NUMBER
1-892693-08-9**

LIBRARY OF CONGRESS CATALOGING IN PUBLICATION DATA
Published in the United States
by
HUGHES HENSHAW PUBLICATIONS
7196 W. 4th Avenue
Lakewood, CO 80226 USA
(303) 237-5905
email: hugheshens@aol.com
www.hugheshenshaw.com

Cover Illustration
David Lee Nutter

Book Cover Design
Dawn Vernon

IMPORTANT INFORMATION

In this book are updated questions and answers that were asked on the National Certification Exam given May 20th, 2000. They include all the modalities listed on the back cover of the book. For those of you who have attended an AMTA Massage Certified School AND you were not taught the Oriental Modalities or other questions that were given on the National Exam, it is very important that you complain to the Administration of your AMTA school because the American Massage Therapy Association is linked with the National Certification Board that gives the National Exam. All the subjects that are being asked on the National Certification Exam should be taught in the AMTA schools since some of the board members on the National Certification Board are associated with the AMTA organization. Some of the individuals who compile the questions for the National Exam are also associated with the AMTA organization. This situation will continue as long as the students don't complain, and demand that this situation be remedied. Our company pioneered the Massage National Exam Questions and Answers book and has been in touch on a monthly basis with students who have just completed taking their National Exam and they email, fax, and overnight letters to us giving us the questions they had on their exams that they did not find in our book, and we compensate them for their efforts as they want future students to be aware of what is being given on this exam. If you have any questions on your exam that you did not find in this book, please notify us as soon as possible and we will financially compensate you immediately. You can contact us at the following addresses and phone/fax numbers:

Hughes Henshaw Publication

7196 West Fourth Avenue - Lakewood, CO 80226-1642

(303) 237-5905 Office 8:00 a.m. - 5:30 p.m. Pacific Time Zone

(303) 233-6545 FAX

emails: hugheshenshaw@home.com and hugheshens@aol.com

www.hugheshenshaw.com

(Currently under construction & being updated)

SECTION I
TEST QUESTIONS AND ANSWERS

1. According to Oriental medicine, what are the three causes of disease?

    Internal (emotions)
    external (the weather and pollution)
    other causes such as germs, poisons, trauma, diet and the effects of drugs.

2. What are two other names for Meridians?

    Channels and pathways, meridians are pathways which life force energy travels

3. Name some of the benefits of yoga.

    Helps circulation, tones muscles and organs, encourages respiration, promotes energy and vitality

4. How many major Meridians are there?

    12

5. In acupressure, what are the gateways to the Meridians?

    The pressure points

6. What are tsubos?

    Another name for pressure points, points on the body that connect meridians, and an area of concentrated energy along a meridian

7. There are three techniques for stimulating the pressure points and they all work to restore the equilibrium and strengthen the flow of Qi or Chi. Name these three.

    Toning - dispersing - calming

8. True or False. You should use ALL pressure points on people who have High and Low Blood Pressure.

    FALSE

9. True or False. You can use ALL pressure points during pregnancy as it helps the unborn child.

    FALSE

10. When you are working on more than one Meridian in a treatment, is it necessary to open one Meridian at a time?

    NO. Do what is most comfortable for you and your patient.

11. True or False. Therapeutic Touch is a massage procedure that applies a very deep pressure working around the connective tissue that wraps around the muscles.

    FALSE. That would be Rolfing.

12. Name 3 techniques used in Hatha Yoga.

    Breathing & relaxing, various body positions, mental concentration, muscle control

13. Why would sports/athletic massage be beneficial after a sporting event?

   It helps to remove toxins stored in the tissues and restores flexibility and mobility and helps to reduce the chance of injuries

14. Name 4 possible negative effects of exercise in sports/athletic massage.

   strains in connective tissue or in the muscle, an increase of metabolic waste build-up in tissues, spasms that restrict movement, inflammation and analogous fibrosis

15. In sports/athletic massage name one reason why deep pressure is used?

   used to deactivate trigger points and relieve stress points

16. What is the longest, main meridian on the back?

   bladder meridian

17. What type of energy is associated with toning, calming, and dispersing?

   TONING is associated with weak energy and when you are toning you use an incense stick which warms the area (the point) and you hold the stick approx. 2cm from the point. Also to tonify at a pressure point you would hold a stationary pressure for approximately 2 minutes. CALMING - you would use your palm to cover the point for approximately 2 minutes

> **DISPERSING** - to disperse energy (Qi) at a pressure point, apply moving pressure with your thumb or fingertip in a circular motion, or *pumping* in and out of the point, for about 2 minutes as this encourages the smooth flow of Qi along the Channels/Meridians.

18. What are the four primary tools used in muscular/structural balancing?

    deep pressure, passive positioning, precision muscle testing and directional massage

19. Where are myofascial trigger points found?

    Located in a tight band of muscle fibers and are found in muscle tissue or associated fascia

20. Name at least 10 benefits of receiving massage therapy.

    improves body alignment
    helps in the process of elimination of waste material
    improves the oxygen supply to cells
    improves relaxation of abdominal and intestinal muscles
    helps to relieve tension
    helps to relieve sore, stiff joints
    helps in the reduction of adhesions, and fibrosis
    helps the nervous system
    helps to relieve insomnia

21. Do most therapists massage by muscle groups?

    Yes, however, it is not mandatory but highly suggested.

22. Name two characteristics of nervous tissue.

    Irritability and conductivity

23. What is Ayurveda?

    It is the ancient healing system of India, and incorporates the triad: body, mind and soul, and consciousness which manifests as earth, air, fire, water and space and believes illness is an imbalance of body systems that can be revealed by taking the pulse and also by examining the tongue.

24. In India's Ayurveda healing treatments and applications, what are the three doshas?

    Vata, pitta, kapha (sometimes referred to as the tri-doshas)

25. Name the functions of each of the doshas: vata, pitta, and kapha.

    VATA- Bodily air, the subtle energy that governs biological movement/breathing
    PITTA - Bodily heat/energy, that governs digestion, absorption, metabolism, body temperature, assimilation, and nutrition
    KAPHA - Bodily stability, maintains body resistance, lubricates the joints, provides moisture to the skin, helps to heal wounds, supports memory retention

26. There are pressure points that you should **NEVER USE** on people who have high or low blood pressure and on people who are pregnant. What are these points and where are they located?

   L14 - Located on the back of the hand in the web between the index finger and the thumb
   B60 - Located on the outside of the ankle between the ankle bone and the Achilles tendon
   SP6- 4 finger widths above the inside ankle bone, just behind the tibia (never use during pregnancy
   K1 - Kidney 1 - you will find this point in the crease in the middle of the ball of the foot, where the color changes from the ball to the sole. Tonify with your elbow to stimulate the kidney Yin and to revive consciousness but NEVER use this point if the client has low blood pressure.

27. What oils and herbs should you never use during pregnancy?

   Marjoram, basil, marigold, myrrh or rue oils and NEVER USE bayberry, motherwort or devil's claw

28. Where is governing vessel (GV20) located and when would you never use this point in a treatment?

   The GV20 is located in the middle of the top of the head between the ears. You would NEVER USE THIS POINT if the client has high or low blood pressure.

29. What are some of the benefits of using various oils in Arvada healing treatments?

Softens the skin, reduces stress, calms the nervous system, and increases the suppleness of the skin.

30. What are two inhibitory reflexes utilized in **M**uscle **E**nergy **T**echnique (MET) ?

Reciprocal inhibition and post isometric relaxation

31. Pertaining to our body, what would be our first line of defense?

The skin

32. If you are having a session and the client wants mostly friction application, would you use a lot of oils and lubricants for friction techniques?

NO, oil reduces friction

33. If you are studying oriental and eastern modalities, you may be asked the following: what marma point helps with leg pains and sciatica?

The sprig point

34. What are marma points?

They are referred to as pressure points in Ayurveda healing.

35. What is another word meaning vascular headaches?

Migraines

36. When you stretch the Achilles tendon, it would increase the flexibility in what part of the body?

Dorsiflexion of the ankle

37. What do the initials ICE and RICE stand for?

ice, compression, and elevation
rest, ice, compression and elevation

38. Yin/Yang is a philosophy about achieving what?

Balance

39. Points near the ends of a meridian are often the most powerful in removing what?

Blocks and in relieving pain along the course of that meridian

40. What are the seven fundamental lessons in Anma?

   1. **massage is not just about understanding techniques but polishing techniques as well**
   2. **do not proclaim yourself as the 'healer.' Establish a rapport with your client.**
   3. **learn to see the body through the hands and not just through the eyes and always give Anma from Tan Den (the area just beneath the navel where**

the center of Ki (universal energy) is. It's very important to know how to breathe properly when working on a client.

4. do not use your intuition to make judgements until you've developed enough fundamental skills
5. "imagination is more important than knowledge." Be cautious but don't be afraid.
6. always follow the flow of Tao (the way of nature), do not work against it.
7. Center and balance yourself by harmonizing Yin and Yang.

41. Name the endocrine glands and the hormones they secrete.

Testes = testosterone
parathyroids = parathormone
corpus luteum in the ovaries = progesterone
ovarian follicle = estrogens
thyroid gland = thyroid hormone [thyroxine and
        triiodothyronine]
pancreatic islets = insulin and glucagon
anterior pituitary = secretes 6 hormones: ACTH, TSH,
        FSH, GH, LH and Lactogenic hormone
adrenal medulla = epinephrine and norepinephrine
posterior pituitary = ADH and oxytocin
adrenal cortex = sex hormones, aldosterone and cortisol

42. If a client complained of shooting pains along the dermatome, numbness or reduced sensation and parenthesis, what could this be a symptom of?

Sciatica, the inflammation of the sciatica nerve.

43. What does the word *Shiatsu* mean?

Finger Pressure and it is a Japanese technique used to treat some illnesses and pain

44. Boils are primarily associated with what type of bacteria?

Staphylococcus

45. In massage of the lower extremity, is the patient usually turned from back-lying to face-lying?

It really depends on whether the patient prefers being massaged on the back first. The patient is not usually turned unless pathologic conditions are such that it seems best to do so

46. If a client has hypertension and complains of being unable to sleep, what treatment would you apply?

1ˢᵗ, massage the neck and the back followed by total body massage, and a general light effleurage touch.

47. A client has had severe arthritis of the whole body for several years and there is a limitation of motion in her left knee; no motion of the patella; and a flexion of deformity of the knee at 145 degrees; what would your treatment be?

You would give her a massage to mobilize the left knee.

48. It is necessary for the student of Oriental Medicine to first study the theory of the Meridian System. It is as important as the student of Western Medicine having to first learn, anatomy, physiology, and pathology.

The 12 regular Meridians (Channels) are listed in the order of vital energy and nutrient flow, with rare exceptions. Please list them.

1.   **Lung (L)**
2.   **Large Intestine (LI)**
3.   **Stomach (St)**
4.   **Spleen (Sp.)**
5.   **Heart (H)**
6.   **Small Intestine (SI)**
7.   **Urinary Bladder (UB)**
8.   **Kidney (K)**
9.   **Pericardium (P)**
10. **Triple Warmer (TW)**
11. **Gall Bladder (GB)**
12. **Liver (Liv)**

49.   Meridians are named according to (1) the organ that is controlled by the energy flow, i.e. lungs, stomach, spleen; (2) the function of the energy, i.e., GV, Regulating Channel (RC), and Motility Channel (MC); and (3) Yin or Yang. In a Yin Meridian, energy mainly flows where?

The location of the Yin Meridians is anterior, therefore it would flow outside.

50.   Name two therapies that are used to release energy.

Polarity therapies and Shiatsu

51.   What are the Yin organs?

Lungs, kidneys, liver, spleen and heart

52. In Shiatsu, where is hara located?

In the abdomen

53. In Ayurvedic assessment, what are the five methods of acquiring information?

Academic, direct   perception and inference, questioning, observation and tactile perception

54. What are marmas?

Ayurvedic energy points

55. What are considered to be the two oldest and most foundational of the healing techniques?

Anma and Ayurveda

56. Are Yin and Yang opposite forces or are they both positive?

Opposite forces

57. Reiki is based on the principles of Chi. What is another name for Chi?

Energy

58. What is the difference between isometric and isotonic?

ISOMETRIC means= of equal dimensions, when the force of the contraction is equal to the resistance i.e.

when the ends of a contracting muscle are held fixed so that contraction produces increased tension at a constant overall length.
ISOTONIC means= having equal tension, denoting the condition when a contracting muscle shortens against a constant load, as when lifting a weight and when the force of the contraction is different from the resistance and movement occurs

59. What is Polarity Therapy based on?

A balanced flow of energy in the body is one of the most important elements for maintaining a healthy body

60. Name a benefit of Therapeutic Touch.

Relieves pain and stress and balances the body's energy by applying a light gentle pressure thereby helping the muscles to contract

61. What does Chelation Therapy do?

Removes toxins

62. Name, in order, the layers of the skin from superficial to deep.

Epidermis, dermis, superficial fascia

63. Define Rolfing.

Rolfing uses deep pressure and manipulation to the connective tissue that helps to restore the alignment of the body

64. Define Reiki.

It is an ancient healing technique that originated from Tibet and uses a very light hand touch on key areas of the body to channel energy to those areas providing a healing sensation or feeling of energy on those areas

65. In oriental modalities the two vessels which travel along the median line on the front and the back are the two most often used for treatment. What are the 2 names and what type of energy is associated with each?

Conception vessel > reservoir of YIN energy
Governing vessel > reservoir of YANG energy

66. _____ is an acupoint or acupuncture point on the body that can be used for relieving pain or to produce certain effects to the internal organs and/or to relieve symptoms.

TSUBO

67. What are the three most modern massage methods based on Anma?

Swedish, Shiatsu, and Tui-na

68. Name at least five contraindications for Shiatsu or Anma.

1. **cancer of leukemia; it can spread if you do massage**
2. **fever**
3. **if client has suffered from an injury or a trauma within 24 hours**

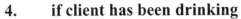

4. **if client has been drinking**
5. **if client has had surgery recently**

69. What consists of the eight-fold examination in Ayurvedic assessment?

   Pulse, tongue, voice, palpation, eyes, form, urine and feces

70. What massage technique is used more than any other in the western world?

   Swedish Massage

71. Name three techniques used in Oriental massage practice.

   Touching, listening, and asking questions

72. Organs receive their autonomic nerve supply primarily from what?

   The homolateral part of the nervous system.

73. What is Qigong?

   Qigong is vital energy of the body. Gong is the skill of working with qi (energy) and it consists of physical movements and breathing exercises for the purpose of improving health and for healing.

74. In Arvada healing what is another name for energy nerves?

   Nadis

75. Tsubos are also referred to as _____ in the West.

   Trigger points

76. Name at least three theories/methods that can be added to enhance the practice of Anma.

   Yin and Yang, five elements theory and tsubo

77. What is Kei Ketsu?

   Tsubo on the meridians directly connected to individual internal organs and supports their functioning

78. List at least 11 contraindications in massage.

   Broken skin, lesions covered by a scab/s, person under the influence of alcohol, cysts, blood clots, warts, varicose veins, ulcers, hematoma, herpes simplex, hives.

79. What is another name for heel-spur syndrome?

   Plantar Fasciitis

80. What is Pancha Karma?

   It is a term used in Ayurveda Healing from India meaning the purification and rejuvenation of the body, mind and soul.

81. In addition to applying pressure on marma points, what else is applied to these points?

   Various essential oils

82. What marma point sends energy to the colon, reproductive organs and bladder?

It is the *oorvee point*

83. What does the word Yoga mean?

Union of the body, mind and spirit, sometimes referred to as union with God

84. List at least 3 different types of fungal infections of the skin.

Jock itch, Athlete's foot, Ringworm

85. What is periostal massage?

It is a technique using trigger points that helps eliminate pain and delay development of the degenerative process in the joints bringing about pathological changes in the periosteum

86. What are some of the contributing factors to insomnia?

Stress, anxiety, physical pain and depression

87. What stroke is generally used when changing from one stroke to another?

The effleurage is sometimes referred to as a transition stroke.

88. The most important thing you can do for your client, in order to maintain a professional relationship, is to be an excellent listener and keep all conversations confidential. Is this true or false?

   True

89. If you were to apply heavy pressure at the back of the knee and massage improperly, what nerve would become entrapped?

   Peroneal Nerve

90. What does TMJ stand for?

   Temporomandibular Joint Disorders

91. It is extremely important to know the endangerment sites on the body because of the possibility of injuring a client. What are some of these sites and where are they located?

   **Upper part of the abdomen under the ribs - abdomen
   axilla is the armpit where there are many nerves
   interior of the ear - notch posterior to the ramus of the
        mandible
   femoral triangle - bordered by the adductor longus
        muscle,
   the inguinal ligament, and the sartorius muscle-
   groin femoral artery
   popliteal fossa - posterior aspect of the knee
   upper lumbar area - lateral to the spine and inferior to
        the ribs
   ulnar notch of the elbow - referred to as the funny bone**

cubital area of the elbow - anterior bend of the elbow
anterior triangle of the neck - bordered by the trachea,
sternocleidomastoid muscle and the mandible-
carotid artery
posterior triangle of the neck - bordered by the clavicle,
trapezius muscle, and the sternocleidomastoid
muscle

92.   What is psychotherapeutic massage?

**An alternative method for the treatment of stress
utilizing both psychology and massage modalities by a
practitioner**

93.   It is very important to set boundaries in your own life and in
your practice. What is one important thing you should not
do?

**You should never combine your massage therapy with
counseling UNLESS you are a registered psychotherapist
and massage therapist. Then the alternative
(psychotherpeutic massage) would be used if you have the
proper credentials and you and your client have
discussed the procedure you would be using.**

94.   Name some of the factors contributing to the formation of
our personal values.

**Significant relationships with others, nature, spirit and
God, meaningful experiences and life changing events.**

95.   What muscles attach to the carocoid process?

Biceps, pectoralis minor, coracobrachalis

96. What is the difference between tendinitis and tenosynovitis?

   Tendinitis is the inflammation of a tendon. Tenosynovitis is the inflammation of a tendon and surrounding synovial sheath.

97. What is the most *non-invasive* form of bodywork?

   Therapeutic Touch

98. What is Anma?

   In Japanese it means = The art of Japanese Massage. It refers to the oldest known form of traditional Asian massage and involves stretching, squeezing, massaging and stimulating the body.

99. When you are taking a client's history, what does the abbreviation SOAP stand for?

   <u>S</u>ubjective findings, <u>O</u>bjective Findings, <u>A</u>ssessment, and <u>P</u>lan.

100. When a new client schedules an appointment, it is important for the body worker to have their client fill out an *intake form* in order to assess their client's needs and any unusual conditions. It lets them know what type of services you offer, just as you would complete a form when going to your medical doctor for the first visit. What are some of the questions & info you should have on your intake form?

Your credentials -
boxes where the client can make check marks √ to
   indicate
yes or *no* **to certain questions ---- questions i.e.:**
What are you wanting to gain from body work sessions?
Are you have any problems? Have you recently
experienced any major emotional, psychological changes,
past traumas? Where do you hold your tension?
It is important to have a very detailed intake form.
Those are just some of the questions you should have on
your form.

101. The word acupuncture combines two Latin words. What are they?

   Acus=needle   and   Punctura=pricking

102. In Oriental Medicine what is the gathering of energy called?

   Research the answer to this question

103. What is the definition of a chakra?

   A wheel of energy

104. What can cause irritation of the sciatic nerve?

   Spasms in the periformis

105. Is it contraindicated to massage a client with encephalitis?

   Yes, if in acute stages

106. What is one purpose of elevating a limb?

To relieve pressure

107. What is another name for a stiff neck?

Torticollis

108. What is the proper response to a client who reports depression and suicidal thoughts during a session?

Refer them to a mental health practitioner

109. Name one result of stress.

Decreased immunity

110. Is the sexual preference of your client considered confidential information?

Yes

111. Jin Shin Do is a form of acupressure that works by releasing what?

Two points simultaneously

112. What constitutes an endangerment site?

It is where you would compress blood vessels or nerves

113. What accommodation might be made during a session for a client with cystitis?

Frequent bathroom breaks

114. When a client does not want to disrobe, what should a massage therapist say?

      They will work through the clothing

115. Is diaper draping a termed used only for infant massage?

      NO

116. What is one of the first things a massage therapist does just before beginning a massage session?

      Wash their hands

117. Client records are confidential except when....?

      by a subpoena or directed by the client

118. What feeling is a client having if a massage therapist observes short, quick breaths and rapid heartbeat?

      Anxiety

119. Be sure and know the 4 stages of rehabilitation.

      Calm spasms - restore flexibility - restore strength restore endurance

120. What is the definition of Kinesiology?

      Study of body movement

121. If you shake your arm or leg what is one result you might obtain?

    Relaxed muscles

122. How much income is reportable to the IRS?

    All of it

123. Sleep deprivation has some consequences. Name at least three.

    Slow healing processes, fatigue, reduced mental capacity

124. What is lordosis?

    Exaggerated concave curve of the lumbar spine

125. What is one way to insure a successful massage practice?

    Have a diversified clientele

126. It is important for the massage therapist to use their body weight when applying certain massage movements. What is considered to be the center of gravity for massage therapists?

    The pelvis

127. Why do most businesses fail?

    Under estimate of capital and expenses

128. Which leg muscles are shortened by wearing high heel shoes?

   Gastrocnemius and soleus

129. What organ is protected by the ribs and sternum?

   Heart

130. If a client came to you and they recently had major surgery, should you give them a massage? What would be a reason/s why your should be cautious?

   Massage can be excellent after surgery BUT DO NOT massage an individual who is on immunosuppressant drugs or who has blood clots. Immunosuppressant drugs are associated with patients who've had cancer surgery or organ transplants. Wait until they are off of their drugs and have, in writing from their physician, permission for massage.

131. What are the sensory receptors that are stimulated during a contract/relax exercise?

   Propriceptors

132. In your first interview with a potential client, should you determine if they have a condition/s that would be contraindicated for massage?

   Yes

133. What is asepsis?

The absence of pathogens

134. What muscle is referred to as the bench-press muscle?

The pectoralis major

135. How would you define CFS (Chronic Fatigue Syndrome)?

A dysfunction of the immune system and can be accompanied by swollen nodes, non-restorative sleep, muscle/joint aches and other symptoms.

136. Alcoholism is considered, by some, to be a disease. If you were to diagnosis alcoholism list at least 4 indications.

memory loss - solitary drinking - neglect of personal responsibilities and use it to feel *normal*

137. Define substance abuse.

Substance abuse is using any substance in dosages or in ways that were not intended to be used by the product or item i.e. food, caffeine, cigarettes, cigars, drugs (prescriptions and illegal ones)

138. What is the definition and function of the lymphatic system?

The lymphatic system includes the lymph, lymph nodes, lacteals, glands, lymph ducts, and lymphatic. The thymus gland, tonsils, and the spleen are also a part of

the lymph system. The function of the lymphatic system is to collect excess tissue fluid invading micro-organisms, damaged
cells and protein molecules. Also the lymphoid tissue produces lymphocytes (a white blood cell) that is an important part of the body's immune system.

139. What is the endangerment site in the inguinal area?

Femoral triangle

140. What is the endangerment site in the anterior neck?

Carotid artery, internal jugular vein, vagus nerve, and the lymph nodes

141. What are the tender spots on muscle tissues called that can emit pain to other parts of the body?

Trigger points

142. If you are massaging a client who has varicose veins, massage would be contraindicated distal or medial to the area of the varicose veins?

Distal

143. What are the boney landmarks where the sciatic nerve passes through the hip?

Ischial tuberosity and the greater trochanter of the femur, bony knob at the top of the leg bone

144. What are the landmarks for locating the brachial plexus?

It is the region between the elbow and the shoulder

145. What is an example of unethical behavior?

Talking about one client's problems to another client

146. What kind of insurance covers hurting a client during a massage?

Malpractice insurance

147. What is the most important skill during client intake?

Listening

148. When you are massaging the upper aspect of the pectoralis major, what endangerment site must you avoid?

Subclavian artery

149. What is edema?

Retention of interstitial fluid due to protein or electrolyte imbalances or due to obstruction in the lymphatic or circulatory systems

150. Would massage be contraindicated in edema?

Yes, if edema is the result of protein imbalance due to breakdown in the kidneys or liver

No, if edema is the result of back pressure in the veins due to immobility

151. Yes or No. If you massage distal to proximal in the lower limbs, would that decrease edema in the lymphatic vessels?

    Yes

152. Would massage be contraindicated for a hematoma?

    Yes

153. Where would a client report discomfort if they had diverticulitis?

    colon

154. What stroke would assist in removing waste from the muscles?

    The kneading stroke

155. How do you recognize varicose veins?

    Lumpy skin, purplish color

156. How do you work with varicose veins?

    Massage proximal to the affected area might be very helpful, especially superficial (barely touching) techniques. Never do a deep massage on small reddish groupings of broken blood vessels that sometimes surround a small protruding vein.

157. What is an example of an ellipsoid joint?

    Wrist

158. Do radioulnar joints glide?

   No, they rotate.

159. Golgi tendon apparatus inhibits what?

   Muscle contraction

160. Does moist heat bring blood to the surface quickly?

   Yes

161. Why would you have a client breathe into their abdomen after an emotional release?

   It activates the parasympathetic nervous system

162. What does the term "window period" mean in reference to HIV?

   It refers to the time between infection and before antibodies can be detected in the blood

163. Is HIV a blood borne pathogen?

   Yes

164. Yes or No. Does HIV die quickly outside of the body?

   Yes

165. Can hepatitis B live outside of the body for up to 3 or more months?

   Yes

166. Does HIV live outside of the for up to 3 or more months?

No

167. Bells Palsy is related to which cranial nerve?

The 7th

168. What dorsiflexes and inverts the foot?

Gastrocnemius

169. What are some of the things that Aromatherapy consists of?

Breathing in or applying essential oils distilled from plants for therapeutic, aesthetic or psychological purposes to heap treat conditions and diseases

170. What is the origin of the short head of the biceps brachii?

The coracoid process

171. What type of joints are found along the spine?

Gliding

172. Why do massage therapists not work directly above pubic symphysis?

That is where the bladder is located

173. Which organ stores bile?

Gallbladder

174. What bodywork movement is used to break down the adhesion of a scar that is well healed?

    Friction

175. What emotion is associated with the gallbladder?

    Anger - you can remember this by saying... "that just galls me"

176. What emotion is associated with the kidneys?

    Fear

177. What emotion is associated with the heart?

    Joy+mental shock

178. What emotions are associated with the spleen energy and lungs?

    Over thinking and worry

179. What are the bony landmarks used to locate the proximal end of the ulna?

    Olecranon process

180. What does the ulna articulate with?

    The head of the radius and humerus above and with the radius below

181. Is the iliopsoas a flexor of the hip?

    Yes

182. What should a massage therapist refrain from wearing while working?

    Strong cologne or perfumes

183. Name the 3 classifications of joints in order of greater to least degree of mobility.

    Diarthrosis, amphiarthrosis, and then synarthrosis

184. Does extension increase or decrease the size of the angle between articulating bones?

    Increases

185. Where do you place the cushion for a client who is lying prone and has lordosis?

    Under the abdomen

186. What is the definition of vasodilation and would friction or kneading cause vasodilation?

    Vasodilation is the widening of the lumen (the space in the interior of a tubular structure such as an artery)of blood vessels and YES friction and/or kneading could cause local vasodilation

187. How do you position a pregnant woman during treatment?

    Lying on her side

188. If a client's legs are uneven where else might you find unevenness?

   In the shoulders

189. What muscles are involved in the flexion of the humerus?

   The pectoralis major, anterior deltoid, and the coracobrachialis

190. True or False. Deep effeurage encourages venous and lymphatic flow.

   TRUE

191. How do you massage a client with osteoarthritis in the neck: how do you massage them?

   Light digital pressure along the cervical vertebrae

192. Define bursa sac and tell where they can be found.

   bursa sac is generally found in connective tissue chiefly about joints and lined with synovial membrane to reduce friction and is found between tendons and bony prominences and other places where there is excessive friction

193. What is the definition of hemopoiesis?

   It is the formation of red blood corpuscles or blood cell formation

194. What flexes the hip and extends the knee?

   The quadriceps

195. Is walking recommended in order to prevent osteoporosis?

   YES

196. Is the pubic symphysis a bony landmark on the anterior pelvis girdle?

   YES

197. What is the definition of isotonic?

   Having equal tension; solutions possessing the same osmotic pressure, more specifically, limited to solution in which cells neither swell nor shrink

198. If a client complains of suffering from constipation, where would the discomfort most likely be?

   Sigmoid colon

199. In oriental medicine which pulse is used for diagnosis?

   Radial pulse

200. A client who is interested in energy work could be referred to whom?

   A reiki practitioner

201. What are some functions of the integumentary system?

Heat regulation, secretion and excretion, sensation, respiration and protection

202. What is the function of ligaments?

To stabilize joints

203. When assessing a range of motion, what are the three things that you examine or observe?

Passisve and active movement and restricted movement First you would perform the active movements, then the passive movements, and then the resisted movements

204. Why do massage therapists take client histories?

to determine if there are any contraindication to massage

205. What is the best way to gather information about a client's complaints?

Observation and palpation

206. Define palpation.

Examination with the hands, feeling for organs, masses, or infiltration of a part of the body, liver, pulse beat; feeling, perceiving by the sense of touch

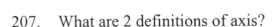

207. What are 2 definitions of axis?

    Vertebral column, the second cervical vertebra

208. What is the atlas?

    First cervical vertebrae

209. How do you stretch the pectoral muscles?

    Abduction and lateral rotation

210. Which stroke encompasses skin rolling?

    Kneading

211. Which stroke is defined as a slight trembling of the hand?

    Vibration

212. What could possible cause a client(while receiving a massage)to have an increase of heart rate and respiration?

    The client could have a memory recollection that had caused them to become anxious/fearful and the heart and respiration increase could be a physiological result of their anxiety.

213. Define Reflexology therapy and Neuromuscular therapy.

Neuromuscular therapy relieves tender muscle tissue and compressed nerves that radiate pain to other areas of the body and reflexology therapy uses certain points on the feet,hands, ankles that correspond to specific organs and tissues in the body and by applying pressure on these points, it can help relieve pain and bring about circulation to the corresponding tissues and organs

214. Define CTS, Carpal Tunnel Syndrome.

It is an irritation of the median nerve as it passes under the traverse carpal ligament into the wrist. It causes numbness, weakness and a tingling sensation. Massage practitioners, court reports, and individuals who use the wrist motion frequently are prone to CTS.

215. Our food passes through the divisions of the large intestine in what order?

Ascending colon > transverse colon > decending colon > sigmoid colon

216. Is a cold application used in the treatment of tendinitis?

YES

217. What is fomentations?

applications of moist heat

218. What is homeostasis?

the state of equilibrium or balance between opposing pressures in the body with respect to various functions and to the chemical compositions of the fluids and tissues. It is also the process through which such bodily equilibrium is maintained, and it is a modern scientific term that happens to describe quite suitably the flow of Ki within and among the meridians. The idea behind *homeostasis* is that dynamic systems (in this case the human body) naturally seek and maintain a condition of overall balance. Whenever an external force is applied to the system, at least one change must occur in the system in order to establish a new condition of balance.

219. What is the first thing you would do if someone is having the symptoms of a heart attack?

    Make them as comfortable as possible (see section on Cardiovascular System in MASSAGE EXAMS, NATIONAL AND STATE BOARD CERTIFICATION QUESTIONS AND ANSWERS, ISBN 0-9617223-1-2)

220. To help remove toxins and waste products from the body, what stroke would be the best to apply?

    Kneading stroke

221. Define *Resisted Exercise*.

    It is the activity of inhibiting muscle contractions initiated by the client.

222. What 3 things/symptoms can appear when a client has a flair-up of Gout?

    Area becomes painful, hot and swollen

223.   Why is lymphatic massage good for sinusitis?

It drains congestion

224.   What strokes are good for bronchitis?

Tapotment

225.   The purpose of Shiatsu is to effect changes in the flow of energy in a meridian by manipulating the energy vortices called _____?

Tsubos

226.   Four primary principles govern Shiatsu techniques. What are they?

1.   **The giver maintains the attitude of an observer.**
2.   **Penetration is perpendicular to the surface of the meridian being treated.**
3.   **Body weight rather than strength is used to allow the hand to penetrate into the meridian that is being worked on.**
4.   **Pressure is applied rhythmically.**

227.   Define a herniated disc.

When a disc is herniated the surrounding annulus fibrosis of an intervertebral disc protrudes and puts pressure on the spinal cord or on nerve roots.

228. Is the fluid which flows into lymph capillaries derived from white blood cells or from blood plasma?

Blood Plasma

229. Name one type of bodywork therapy would help release the flow of energy through the body.

Polarity

230. Some contraindications exist when using finger pressure to acupuncture points. Where would you avoid using finger pressure?

Directly over contusions, scar tissue or infection, or if the patient has a serious cardiac condition, pregnancy and high or low blood pressure, and children under 7 years of age should not be treated with these techniques.

231. What is the first symptom that one gets when they are afflicted with osteoarthritis?

Burning, stinging, sharp pain in and around the joints particularly in the hands, knees and hip area

232. When someone is having an epileptic seizure what is the first thing you would do?

Clear the way of any surrounding objects that might be in the way and make it as comfortable for them as possible

233.   Can massage get rid of stretch marks.

        NO

234.   The periformis is a source of sciatic pain when entrapped by what nerve?

        Sciatic nerve

235.   There are several abbreviations that are asked on your exams.   RESEARCH THESE.

ROM	**= Range of Motion**
ANS	**= Autonomic Nervous System**
CNS	**= Central Nervous System**
COPD	**= Chronic obstructive pulmonary disease**
ATP	**= Adenosine 5'-triphosphate**
PCP	**= phencyclidine**
AIDS	**= acquired immunodeficiency syndrome**
CPR	**= cardiopulmonary resuscitation**
ELISA	**= enzyme-linked immunoadsorbent assay**
HIV	**= human immunodeficiency virus**
HBV	**= hepatitis B virus**
EDTA	**= ethylenediaminetetraacetic acid (edathamil, acid)**
TMJ	**= temporomandibular joint (dysfunction)**
SOAP	**= subjective (data), objective (data), assessment, and plan (problem-**

236.   What are two *possible* signs of AIDS in the early stages?

        Night sweats and chronic diarrhea

237. Is it a good idea to consider, in AIDS prevention, that all body fluids that are wet could possibly be contaminated?

    YES

238. The following case is being used to illustrate possible choices that can be made using combinations of techniques from three popular systems, namely *Swedish Massage, Shiatsu, and Polarity (information from Beverly Kitss, R.P.T.)* There is also some additional consideration given for this case. One intention in showing a sample case is to indicate how well different methods can integrate with one another. The case also offers pointers for expanding the number of choices and possibilities for practice. It is meant to encourage exploration in the application of methods. The case is not meant to offer stock formulas, as there is no way of knowing how to respond until one is actually present with the client.

CASE: Client: GENERAL FATIGUE

A 37-year-old woman complains of fatigue and irritability since the recent holiday season. She feels that she has been caring for everyone's needs but her own, and now she wants to give herself a gift of relaxing massage.

Possible Session

Swedish Massage: give general relaxing Swedish massage with special attention to areas of tension. *Polarity:* intersperse Polarity techniques with Swedish massage for stimulating parasympathetic nervous system, thus deepening the state of relaxation. *Shiatsu:* work feet and hands.

Additional Considerations

Each of our three sample systems has elements that can help bring forth the most relaxed response to the work. In Swedish massage, the tempo and rhythm of stroking and kneading often add to the comfort and relaxation of the patient. In the same way, the Polarity practitioner may use rhythmical oscillations and gentle holding. The Shiatsu practitioner may seek a rhythm harmonizing the pressure and release with the breathing of the receiver.

The voice tone of the practitioner may convey certain feelings of warmth and relaxation. There may be a selection of music from which the receiver may choose a piece of special background music. Environmental elements such as heat, lighting, and ventilation should all be checked before starting the session. Be prepared for the possibility that massage may free the patient to express previously suppressed emotions, for this is a common response and may be as therapeutic as the bodywork itself.

239. Name the four basic steps in a therapeutic procedure that would be specific to a client's complaint.

Assessment, Evaluation, Planning, and Performance

240. What is the best manipulation for local deep massage of soft tissue?

Deep effleurage

241. What is the best manipulation for scar tissue?

Friction

242. True or False. Most therapeutic relationships with clients should be Professional.

True. The client feels you can help and are knowledgeable when you act in a professional manner.

243. What style of massage has the most specific touch and direction of touch? Trager, reflexology, rolfing, reike, etc?

Answer: reflexology

244. What structure do you have to be cautious of in the femoral triangle area?

Femoral artery

245. Be sure you know the direction of blood traveling from the left side of the heart throughout the body and back again to the heart i.e.

Right atrium receives blood from large superior and inferior vena cava > from right atrium the venous blood passes through the tricuspid valve into the (r) ventricle > from the (r) ventricle the venous blood is pumped

through the pulmonary semilunar valve and is carried thru the pulmonary arteries to the lungs to be oxygenated > the freshly oxygenated blood is then collected into the capillaries into the pulmonary veins and returned to the heart > the (l) atrium receives the oxygenated blood from the pulmonary veins > from the (l) atrium the oxygenated blood passes thru the mitral valve in the (l) ventricle > the (l) and from the (l) ventricle the blood is pumped thru the aortic semilunar valve and into the aorta > from the aorta the blood is distributed to the major arteries except for the lungs and then the blood moves into smaller branches of the arterial system until it flows into the arterioles > from the arterioles the blood goes into the thin-walled capillaries where the nutrients, fluids and oxygen move into the tissue spaces and CO_2 and wastes are reabsorbed into the blood stream and the blood stream is collected from the capillary beds into the venules and then into larger veins until the blood finally flows into the superior or inferior vena cava > and this cycle is repeated and starts all over again

246.   What muscle is affected with the hiatus hernia?

Diaphragm

247.   **NOTE**: Be sure you know the functions of the skin, the name of the skin, vitamin D synthesis, synthesizes various chemicals, houses sensory receptors, etc.   There are more functions. This has been asked on several exams.

248.   Would Golgi's tendon organ be a sensory end organ?

YES

249.   What is dyspnea?

Shortness of breath or distress in breathing usually associated with disease of the heart or lungs and can occur during intense physical exertion or at high altitude

249.   How is lymph moved through the body?

Flows in the lymphatic vessels through the lymph nodes and is eventually added to the venous blood circulation

250.   In massaging the chest muscles (example: the pectoralis minor or major) where would you place the pillows during the massage?

Under the arms so as to relax the chest muscles

251.   What part of the body would be affected in case of diverticulitis?

The colon. It is inflammation of small pouches (diverticula) that forms on the wall of the colon

251.   **Note:** Know all aspects of first aid procedures and the order in which you would apply first aid i.e. check out the scene, responsiveness, call 911, EMS, tilt head, etc. This is asked on most exams.

252.   Insertion of iliopsoas muscle is what?

Lesser trochanter of femur

253. When you are lying prone, which of the following muscles on the back range from deep to superficial?

erector spinae, serratus posterior, rhomboids, levator scapula, latissimus dorsi, trapezius

254. Stretching, pulling, etc. can help in what condition? Bruising, scar tissue or what?

Scar tissue

255. Patient says that they don't feel well. What would you do?

Study this because there are several examples of why they don't feel well. Know what to do under several circumstances.

256. What is the wrong position for a client to be in with posterior varicose veins in lower legs?

Having a bolster in back of knees and lower legs is a "no no."

257. What are some contraindications for oriental massage?

Choices: terminal illness, serious heart conditions, advanced diabetes

258. Where does the absorption of the most nutrients and fluids take place?

Small intestine

259. Insertion of the biceps femoris is where?

head of fibula

260. What three techniques are used in sports/athletic massage besides those used in Swedish massage?

active joint movements, compression and cross-fiber friction

261. Palpation of the psoas muscle could endanger which structure?

External iliac vein and artery

262. Would the femoral artery be involved with an endangerment site?

YES, it terminates as the popliteal artery

263. What affliction is torticolli and what part of the body is affected?

Wry neck, muscle contraction on one side of neck causing head to be tilted and twisted to one side.

264. Ileocecal valve is between which two structures?

Small and large intestines

265. **Note:** Research why it is important to massage the ileocecal valve and why it is beneficial and how long and how often you should massage this area.

266. In what order is the *"normal way of walking.?"*

Heel, lateral surface, then the toes

267. What is synovitis?

Inflammation of synovial capsule

269. What is the name of the type of scar with excessive tissue build up?

Keloid scar

268. On the anterior medial side of the wrist, which muscle tendons are you palpating?

Flexor carpiulnaris

269. Tidbit of information. Flexors of the humerus (some tests give grouping of muscles to choose from, i.e) ...coracobrachialis, biceps brachi, brachialis, brachioradialis. Know the flexors and the grouping of muscles

270. No pressure should be used around auxiliary area because of the _____?

musculocutaneous nerve

271. What is the best massage stroke to break up area of fibrois (hard tissue build up)?

Friction or deep effleurage

272. If your client suddenly takes a long deep breath and then starts breathing at a slower rate...why would this happen?

     The parasympathetic nervous system has taken over

273. Full rotation in a circular motion of the wrist includes which motion? Pronation, supination or circumduction

     circumduction

274. What is the best manipulation for local deep massage of soft tissue?

     Deep effleurage

275. Static pressure on patient who contracts muscle would be what? Choices are: isometric, isotonic, etc.

     Answer: isometric

278. What does shiatsu, acupuncture, and anma therapy have in common?

     They use pressure points

279. What *system* protects the body, excretes waste, and regulates temperature?

     Integumentary system

280. If you are massaging a client and that client wants you to squeeze a pimple or blackhead, what would you tell the client and why would you not do this?

You should never squeeze a pimple because you could do damage and you could also spread infection.

281. Which stroke would most effectively address *adhesion in tendinous tissue?*

Friction

282. What would describe the effects of fascial adhesions?

Decreased muscle power w/increased chance of injury

283. Which hormone stimulates retention of water by the kidneys?

ADH

284. There are two main classifications of glands. Please name the two glands.

Duct glands/exocrine and the ductless glands/endocrine

285. Which organ is located in the upper right quadrant of the body?

   Liver

286. Which organ is located in the upper left area below the ribs?

   Spleen

287. There are five elements that represent the qualities of ki energy. What are they?

   Wood, metal, water, earth, fire.

288. Which muscle originates at the sacrum, inserts on the greater trochanter, and is an external rotator of the hip?

   Piriformes

289. Abdominal inhalation requires contraction of which of the following muscles?

   Answer: diaphragm

290. What hydrotherapy modality is used to decrease pain and cellular metabolism?

   Ice Pack

291. The mastoid process is an insertion point for what muscles?

    Splenius capitus and the sternocleidomastoid

292. The purpose of the pleural fluid surrounding the lungs is to do what?

    Lubricate the opposed membrane

293. In which abdominal pelvic quadrant is the sigmoid flexure of the colon located?

    Lower left

294. Digested food stuffs or contents are passed through the large intestine in what order?

    Ascending, transverse, descending, and sigmoid colons

295. Which of the following best describes Psoriasis?

    Chronic skin disorder (this appears but the question is worded differently)

296. The muscles of the posterior thigh from lateral to medial are: **Biceps femoris, semitendinosus, and Semimembranosus.**

297.	The parasympathetic system is stimulated by what type of massage stroke?

	Long gliding strokes

298.	Name 6 important endrocrine glands.

	Sex glands (gonads), pituitary gland, parathyroid glands, thyroid gland, pancreas, and adrenal glands.

299.	The structure you are concerned about in the adductors muscle group is which of the following?

	This was on a multiple choice question

300.	Which bone is the lateral malleus associated with?

	This was on a multiple choice question

301.	Of the following which would be a distinguishing factor of rheumatoid arthritis.

	This was on a multiple choice question.

302.	The vertebral artery is vulnerable when doing what manipulation?

When massaging just below the mastoid continuing down the neck. Be careful of endangerment sites.

303. Which are the 2 muscles that move the mandible?

    This was on a multiple choice question

304. How would you treat a client if they had tennis elbow?

    Massage the extensor muscles of the forearm and the lateral epicondyle with cross-fiber friction, compression, deep stroking and soothing effleurage.

305. When you are lying prone, which of the following muscles on the back extend from deep to superficial?

    Deep layer: intercostals, rotattores, multifidus, levatores. Intermediate layer: longissimus, erector spinae, serratus. Superficial layer: Lattissimus dorsi, trapezius, rhomboid

306. If a client happens to fall just prior to coming to see you for their appointment and they injured their ankle and said they were in pain when they moved it, however you notice no swelling or redness, what would you do in this case or what would you suggest?

Do not work directly on the injury. Suggest they wrap the ankle and go see their doctor.

307. If a client comes in complaining of pain in their right shoulder from a car accident, which of the following would be an appropriate response? (A) have you seen a doctor? (B) would you like an Aspirn? (c) did you get the name of the person who hit you? (D) what motion creates pain?

    ANSWER: A&D

308. What structure would be endangered at the ulna humeral area?

    The Ulnar nerve

309. _____tissue lines the surface of the integumentary system?

    Epithelial tissue

310. You would encourage a client to stretch_____muscle if they have Kyphosus.

    Pectoralis major and minor

311.   _____ is a modality that does not involve touching the client's body.

Healing Touch or Therapeutic touch

312.   The modality that uses the tongue, pulse, and hara (breathing) in the assessment is called _____.

Ayurvedic

313.   _____ is the organ that is responsible for filtering old, dead red blood cells.

Spleen

314.   Where does lymph return to circulation?

Subclavian vein

315.   These 3 (perimysium, epimysium, and endomysium) form the structure of what?

Muscle fiber

316.   The sciatic nerve is located where?

Gluteal region, hamstrings and lower leg

317. When palpating the popliteal fossa, the structure to be aware of is which of the following?
(A) tibial nerve
(b) popliteal artery
(c) common peroneal nerve
(d) all of the above

ANSWER: D

318. Tibialis anterior is innervated by _____?

Deep peroneal nerve

319. _____vessel goes from the heart to the lungs?

Pulmonary arteries

320. _____ is appropriate for an acute sprain/strain.

Massage

321. _____is the muscle used during normal, quiet breathing.

The diaphram

322. _____ _____ muscles are used during forceful inspiration.

External intercostals/serratus posterior superior

323. What is the correct order from lateral to medial?
(A) biceps femoris, semitendionous, semimembranosus
(b) sartorius, gracilis, adductor longus
(c) rectus femoris, vastus lateralis, vastus medialis

ANSWER: A

324. _____is where you would place a pillow while working on pectoralis minor.

Underneath abducted bent elbow, lying supine

325. _____ would use scented oils and lotions.

Aromatherapy

326. _____ would be the most appropriate technique that you would apply if a client had spastic colon.

Therapeutic touch/healing touch

327.   What is pes• anserinus?

   Intraparotid plexus of the facial nerve

328.   What principal are you using when you contract a muscle to increase its flexibility?

   PNF Proprioceptive neuromuscular facilitation

329.   Working _____ muscle you increase the flexibility of dorsiflexion.

   Gastrocnemius

330.   You are stimulating _____ when you put one hand on the occiput and the other hand on the sacrum.

   Cerbrospinal fluid motion or craniosacral motion

331.   Fill in the blanks: _____ muscle is palpated between the iliac _____ and the greater trochanter.

   Crest (gluteus medius)

332.   Tennis elbow is best evidenced or indicated by what?
   Inflammation and/or some tenderness of the lateral epicondyle

333.   Which bone does the fibia articulate with at the ankle joint?

Talus

334.   Name another symptom of tennis elbow and another area that could involve tennis elbow.

Painful wrist extensor - also the lateral epicondyle

335.   If you have been massaging a client and you notice that your client stops breathing, and after you have checked for responsiveness to make sure they are not breathing, what would you do next?

Call 911 Immediately.

336.   Should your client, all of a sudden during the massage treatment, tell you they are experiencing some dizziness, complain of some pain down their left arm and some numbness, what is the first thing you would do?

Remain calm, get the client into a comfortable position and call emergency immediately (either 911) OR depending upon your geographical area, the fire department or police dept.

337. When working with the sternocleidomastoid what artery should be avoided?

   Carotid

338. Please define hara breathing.

   hara breathing is when the breaths are directed to the lower abdomen.

339. When you are working with a client and you begin to notice an very *sweet sickening acetone like odor* emitting from their body, what would you do, and what could be one possible cause for this?

   You would suggest they see their physician because it could possibly be a sign of a *diabetic condition* but remember you are *NEVER TO DIAGNOSIS*.

340. If you are massaging a client and your client suggests to you that they would like for you to relieve them sexually, what are some things you can tell your client?

   Remind them the purpose of Massage Therapy and you could also ask your client to leave and if there were problems you should call 911.

341. What is another word for *an unknown cause*.

   Idiopathic

342. Red blood cells are formed in what tissue?

   Myeloid

343. Pressure applied to hands and feet is usually done by a
   _____?

   Reflexologist

344. How often are you to file your Federal Tax Forms?

   Quarterly

345. Why would you want to have Liability Insurance and please
   give an example of what this type of insurance would cover?

   **Liability insurance covers a client falling or becoming
   injured on your property**

346. Why should you *not* place attractive throw rugs in your
   working area?

   Client could trip or fall

347.   What kind of stretching of the muscles can cause harm?

When using MET (Muscle Energy Techniques) the therapist should not use ballistic movements against the contractions when they are working with the client in stretching muscles (passive stretching)

348.   **Note:** On a recent exam (2000) there were four drawings. It read: Please choose the drawing that would be *contraindicated* for a client with varicose veins that are located on the posterior portion of the legs.   Drawing had a bolster under the knee and calf

349.   During a massage session, if your client suddenly recalls an incident of having been sexually abused as a child, what would you do or what would you recommend?

First thing I suggest is not to make a big issue out of it but tell your client this is certainly not an unusual occurrence as this happens sometimes during a massage treatment and suggest they discuss it with their family physician, or seek therapy from a therapist who works with sexually abused persons.

350.   What position would your head be in if your SCM muscles were contracted bilaterally?

The flexion position

351. What type of massage stroke would you use in the mandibular region?

Circular- friction

352. Please describe how to recognize a parasympathetic condition and tell what the general function of the parasympathetic division is.

Watch client's breathing. When it changes and client takes in a deep breath followed by slower quieter breathing, this is the meaning of parasympathetic. The function of the parasympathetic is to calm and to conserve energy and to reverse action of the sympathetic division.

353. If a client complains of pain in the hip area and also some numbness down the leg, what could this indicate?

Sciatica and periformis problems

354. You should be careful of what nerve when working on the sartorius?

Femoral

355. Joint movement is the strongest when the muscle attachment is near what?

Insertion point

356. If your client begins to perspire, this indicates that the _____ system is working?

Sympathetic

357. Other than Swedish Massage Therapy, what other methodology would involve pressure point therapy at specific points while moving the hands and fingers in a specific direction?

Applied Reflex ology

358. If you are massaging a client and they start to have an extreme anxiety attack, with profuse sweating and palpitation, what should you do?

Treat is as an *emergency*.

359. This question was on the exam however, it was worded slightly differently than those in our books. If a client says

they have been diagnosed with a peptic ulcer, what would be one of the things you *would not do?*

You would not apply any pressure on their back.
NOTE: THIS PAGE SKIPPED TO NUMBER 361.
There is no 360.

361.   What is diverticulosis and where would it be located?

Diverticulosis is an inflammation of a sac opening out
from a tubular organ or main cavity and it is located in
the large intestine

362.   When massaging the _____region you should be careful NOT to injure the musculocutaneous nerve.

Auxiliary region. This question has been asked several
different ways on the test.

363.   The _____ and _____ are considered agonist/antagonist?

Biceps brachii and triceps brachii. This questions has
been asked differently on the National also i.e. What pair
of muscles are considered antagonist/agonist?

364.   If a person contracts a muscle and this muscle is pushing against static pressure, what is this considered to be?

Isometric

365. **Note:** In Oriental Medicine YIN is located mainly where? Be sure to brush up on all of your oriental massage questions pertaining to yin, yan, meridians, elements, pulse taking etc. They ask several questions on oriental medicine modalities.

366. One book states Yin is dark|night; cold; inside; while Yan is described as being _____?

    light|day| hot| outside

367. If a client stops breathing and is unresponsive in a supine position, what do you do?

    Call EMS, open airway, give breaths, and check pulse (Standard first aid of course).

368. What is the anterior tendon that is the midway portion of the wrist near the crease and what positions provide a full range of motion for the wrist?

    Tendon of flexor carpi ulnaris and the positions would be: flexion, extension, pronation and supination

369. What organ is involved in the production of white blood cells? This question is also one that is in our study guides however, it is worded differently on some exams.

    The spleen

370. Name a muscle that spans two points.

Gastrocnemius

371. In Oriental Bodywork name the Yin organ that corresponds to the Earth aspect of the world.

The spleen

372. What is the muscle that inverts the foot?

Tibialis anterior

373. In reflex ology, where is the point that corresponds to the neck and head?

Big toe

374. What is the synergist muscle to the periformis?

Gluteus maximus

375. What is the main function of ligaments?

Stabilize joints

376. Why does injured cartilage take so long to heal?

Because it has little blood supply

377. Name the joints of the pelvic girdle.

Hip, sacroiliac & pubic symphysis

378. What is a likely contraindication for massage when massaging a client with diabetes?

Varicosis

379. What extra considerations might you have for someone with hypothyroidism?

May need to increase room temperature

380. What position would you place a client's arm while they are in the supine position when massaging the serratus anterior?

Place pillows under the arms

381. What structure should be avoided when massaging in the axillary region?

Armpit

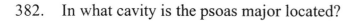

382. In what cavity is the psoas major located?

Abdominal

383. What is Eastern Anatomical position?

Hands above the head

384. How would you give physical support to a client in the supine position who had dowagers hump?

Pillow under head and neck

385. In the five elements of oriental theory, what organ is yang to the earth?

Stomach

386. In the five elements of oriental theory, what organ is yin to the fire element?

Heart NOTE: Brush up on the oriental medicine applications

387. What muscle is a synergist to the piriformis?

Gluteus maximus

388. What two (2) muscles are antagonistic to each other?

Erector spinae and erectis abdominus

389. As a massage|body worker, what would be the best response to a new client who refused to fill out the client intake form?

Choose NOT to take that client. Approximately 100 letters that have been mailed or faxed to our company had this question on their exam.

390. In acupressure the pulse is taken to read the energy fields related to the organs. Where is the sight in which the pulse is taken?

The wrist.

391. Name a bony landmark for the brachial plexus.

Clavicle

392. Name the structure that inhibits muscle contractions.

Neurotendinous organs

393. What kind of neurons pick up information from receptors and send to the brain and spinal cord?

Sensory

394. What kind of bodywork produces emotional releases that are then reinforced with other aspects of the therapy?

Reichian Therapy

395. What is the name of the reddened skin response to massage therapy?

Hyperemia

396. What membrane is stimulated in joint mobilization?
Synovial membrane

397. What kind of joint allows movement in only a single plane?

Hinge joint

398. What organ of the body helps to regulate body temperature?

Skin

399. Which artery is used to take a pulse in oriental bodywork?

Radial

400. Which muscle would you work on if someone complained of patella pain?

   Quadriceps

401. What is the 10th cranial nerve?

   Vagus nerve

402. When massaging near the inguinal ligament what structure would you avoid applying deep pressure to?

   Femoral nerve

403. When applying resistence to the knee while extended the leg, what muscle is the primary mover?

   Vastus intermedius

404. If you notice a regular client has a mole that has increased in size, what would be the best choice of action?

   Tell the client you noticed it and refer your client to a family physician for inspection

405. What structure should you avoid when palpatating the tissue at the insertion of the biceps femoris?

   Common peroneus nerve

406. What countries are represented in TOUCH FOR HEALTH?

   Canada, Mexico, New Zealand, France, Japan, Netherlands, China, Germany, Australia, Puerto Rico

407. What hormone is produced to effect low blood sugar?

   Insulin

408. What is the name of the area of concentrated energy in a meridian line?

   Acupoint or acupuncture points (small areas of high conductivity)

409. What organ mostly controls digestion in oriental bodywork?
   Stomach

410. What are the symptoms of anxiety or having an anxiety attack?

   Very similar to having a heart attack; panic, quick breathing, can't catch your breath

411. A client has informed you that they have HIV and your are uncomfortable working with them, what do you do?

    Acknowledge it, talk it over and come to a mutual agreement

412. In what type of bodywork does the practitioner apply static pressure with a low release and a stretch?

    Neuro-muscular

413. How would a massage/body worker address a client who has a peptic ulcer?

    1st thing to do is ask if they are on any medication; 2nd don't massage around the abdomen area because you don't want to put any pressure near the ulcer nor heavy pressure on the back opposite the ulcer

414. What type of massage technique would you use for a person with constipation?

    Slight massage in clockwise direction over the intestinal areas

415. In what layer of the skin are vessels and nerves found?

    Dermis

416. When a client has Kyphosus, what muscles are contracted?

   Abdominal

417. What is effected when a person has a sprain?

   Ligaments

418. In oriental theory what is YIN and YANG?

   In Buddhist thought they are the two parts that contrast or exist as opposites of the same phenomenon

419. If someone was healing from a soft tissue injury why would you apply massage?

   To reduce the building up of scar tissue

420. A runner has just injured his or her ankle. It is swollen, red, hot, and is beginning to turn black and blue. What would it be considered to be?

   Hematoma

421. What effect does massage have on urine output?

   Has a tendency to increase the output

422. What is dermatome?

A segmental skin area enervated by various spinal cord segments; the lateral portion of the somite of an embryo which gives rise to the dermis of the skin; the cutis plate. ALSO it is referred to as "instrument for incising the skin or for cutting thin transplants of skin.

423. What organ is protected by the vertebral column & sternum?

Heart

424. What is idiopathic?

Cause unknown, no identification for a disease

425. If you sweat, what system is this?

Excretory system

426. Infection from bladder to kidneys: **ureter**

427. What is diverticulosis?

Inflamation of the colon

428. Most of our food is digested where?

Small intestine

429. Where are the adrenal glands located?

Top of kidneys

430. To move the vertebrae in your back, would this be considered flexion and extension?

Yes

431. Where is the gall bladder located.

Upper right quadrant of the body.

432. What are purkinje fibers?

A typical muscle fibers lying beneath endocardium of heart which constitute the impulse-conducting system of the heart

433. What is referred to sometimes as Potts Curve or Kyphosus?

A spinal curvature, an exaggeration or angulation of normal posterior curve of the spine - sometimes referred to as humpback| hunchback| convex curve

434. What does PSIS stand for?

Posterior superior iliac spine area

435. The apical pulse is located where?

Below the left nipple

436. Cold applications are use to do what?

Reduce swelling

437. What is the Heimlich maneuver and why is it used?

It consists of inward and upward thrusts on a person's abdomen between the rib case and navel when a person is choked on a piece of food or other object, it hopefully throws the food of lodged object out of the persons mouth

438. If a client comes to your for a massage and has a stoma, please describe what this is.

It is an opening to a colostomy through which the person empties fecal contents into a bag

439. What is a prosthesis?

A device such as an artificial limb

440. What is the normal range for pulse rate in an adult at rest?

60-90 beats per minute

441. Name the muscles of the back starting from internal to external.

Intercostalis, rhomboids, and trapezes

442. The extenders of the wrist are on the _____?

Lateral condole of the humerus

443. Where is the origin of the wrist Flexors?

Medial condole of humerus

444. If your client suddenly stops breathing what should you do?

Open their airway - give two breaths - call 911

445. What is the tsubo?

Area of concentrated energy along a meridian.

446. Name some reasons applications and reasons they are used in sports/athletic massage.

Deep pressure is used to relieve stress, cross-fiber friction is used to reduce fibrosis, compression is used to create hyperemia in the muscle tissue and active joint movements are used in the rehabilitation of various conditions i.e injuries for rehabilitation of neurologic and soft tissue disorders, for proprioceptive Neuromuscular facilitation (PNF).

447. Which quadrant is the liver located in?

Upper right

448. What would help a client with osteoporosis?

Weight bearing exercises

449. What is above the pubic and is sensitive?

The bladder

450. What type of insurance would cover an injury in your office or your property?

Liability

451. What technique in massage would move one layer of tissue over another?

Friction

452. Rocking and rolling techniques are used in what type of massage?

    Trager

453. What treatment would be used for acute bursitis?

    Ice

454. Shiatsu is associated with what type of pressure?

    Finger pressure

455. Would an ice pack decrease cellular metabolism?

    Yes

456. Give one reason why you would have your client fill out a medical history report?

    To identify areas of indications and contraindications and other areas of concern prior to giving a massage

457. What is the secondary effect of using ice?

    It is to increase or decrease blood flow. Look this up. It is on the National exam

458. Hot or cold would not be used with a person who has _____.

Neurologic impairment

459. What would be the best technique to promote lymphatic flow?

Deep effleurage

460. If a client seems depressed and discusses the thoughts of committing suicide, or happens to remember a childhood sexual abuse incident, what should you do?

Suggest they schedule an appointment with their physician or a counselor who specializes in those issues.

461. How much of the money your receive from your clients should you declare on your taxes/IRS?

All

462. What would the movement be between carpal bones?

Gliding

463. What technique would you use when beginning a massage session?

Effleurage

464. Where is the only saddle joint found in the body?

Your thumb

465. Where does the short head of the biceps brachii originate?

Coracoid process

466. Moist heat pack is contraindicated for the treatment of what?

Edema

467. What artery causes the back of the knee to be an endangerment site?

Popliteal artery

468. _____ churning occurs in the large intestines.

Haustral

469. Where is the mitral valve located?

It is the valve closing the orifice between the L atrium and the L ventricle of the heart.

470. _____is a skin condition that is scaley, flakes off and is usually red.

Psoriasis

471. What position should the client be in when working the iliotibial band?

On side with upper leg slightly bent and supported over the lower leg

472. Is impetigo a contagious skin condition?

Yes

473. Tongue and hara diagnosis are used by what type of bodywork?

Shiatsu

474. What should you avoid when you are doing a power massage?

Inhaling the powder

475. How should the client's arm be positioned when you are working the latisimus dorsi?

The client should be in the prone position with their arm raised by side of head

476. What would you use instead of lotion or oil if your client has greasy skin?

Powder

477. If a client tells you that they are having a problem and needs to have their chakras balanced, who would you refer her to?

A polarity practitioner

478. What acts as the stretch receptor?

Golgi tendon organ

479. Where are the intercostal muscles located?

Between the ribs

480. Name the condition that biofeedback is mostly used for.

Asthma and stress|anxiety

481. When you are working under the clavicle what blood vessels should you avoid?

Subclavian

482. What is a lateral curvature to the spine called?

Scoliosis

483. Cluster headaches and migraine headaches are called what?

Vascular headaches

484. Local application of cold produces what?

Vasoconstriction

485. What are the two most common stances?

Archer and horse stance

486. Contracting the neck flexors bilaterally would result in what?

Lifting the head while in a supine position

487. If a client had chickenpox would this be a contraindication for massage?

Yes

488. What exercise is good to increase flexibility and improve relaxation?

Yoga

489. How would you position your client in order to relax the pectoralis major?

Supine position with pillows under the arms

490. If a client had twisted their ankle before coming to you for a massage session and they were limping and said that it was alright, what should you do?

Refer them to their physician

491. If you are massaging a client and they "get out of hand and become threatening in any manner" what should you do?

Immediately leave your work area and call for professional help, usually 911.

492. During meditation sometimes the _____ system is activated.

Parasympathetic

493. What is a technique that can assess a weakness in a muscle?

Range of Motion ROM or Touch For Health

494. Pain that occurs in one area but originates from another area is called _____?

Referred pain

495. What is ischemia?

Local anemia due to mechanical obstruction of the blood supply

496. Scar formation is called _____?

Fibrosis

497. Where does a strain occur?

In the muscles

498. What muscle is usually involved in *frozen shoulder*?

Subscapularis

499. What organ can be palpated under the right rib?

Liver

500. What should be avoided at the insertion of the biceps femoris?

Common peroneal nerve

501. What is the name of the muscle that works against the prime mover?

Antagonist

502. Where should heavy tapotment be a voided?

Over the chest area and one the back (if a person has an ulcer)

503. What is the name of the movement that occurs when a muscle does not lengthen or shorten?

Look this up. It is on most exams.

504. Specific joint movements are caused by the _____?

Prime mover

505. Recently it was discovered children who are on the drug Ritalin can reduce much of their hypertension by removing sugar and white flour products from their diet.

A tidbit of info

506. What are these two very harmful foods that are making children & adults "hyper active"?

Sugar, any sugar by-products or foods whose name end in "ose" i.e. maltose, dextrose, etc. And white flour and any foods that have white flour by products as an ingredient. Also the movie that Merryl Streep starred in February 16, 1997 on ABC which told about the 2 year old boy who was having 90 epileptic seizures a day and was CURED after his DIET was altered. Research alternative ways to get off of drugs that have very harmful side effects. Usually a change in diet with proper exercise can produce what appears to be a miracle.

507. What is osteoclast and what is it used for?

It is an instrument used to fracture a bone in order to correct a deformity

508. What is keratin?

A scleroprotein or (hard protein) albuminoid (a simple type of protein) present in hair and in nails

509. Name 3 contraindications for hydrotherapy.

Lung disease, infectious skin conditions and kidney infection

510. When the client is in the prone position the soleus muscle is underneath the _____ ?

    Gastrocnemius

511. Name an area where you would NOT perform heavy tapotements?

    On the chest

512. What is a prime mover?

    It is responsible for causing a joint action

513. What is another name for fat tissue?

    Adipose

514. What muscles are used when you grate your teeth, move your jaw and smile?

    Pterygoideus pateralis   and pterygoideus medialis

515. Name two things cold water application improves.

    Stimulates nerves and improves circulation

516. What part of the body should be raised when massaging the abdominal area?

The knees

517. What does compression do?

It pushes muscles against the bones

518. Name 11 endangerment sites and their locations.

Interior of the ear = notch posterior to the ramus of the mandible

Upper lumbar area = just inferior to the ribs and lateral to the spine

Axilla = Armpit

Popliteal fossa = posterior aspect of the knee

anterior triangle of the neck = bordered by the mandible, sternocleiodomastoid muscle and the trachea

abdomen = upper area of the abdomen under the ribs

femoral triangle = bordered by the sartorius muscle, the adductor longus muscle and the inguinal ligament

ulnar notch of the elbow = the funny bone

cubital area of the elbow = anterior bend of the elbow

medial brachium = upper inner arm between the biceps and tricepts

posterior triangle of the neck = bordered by the sternocleidomastoid muscle, the trapezius muscle and the clavicle

519. Name the six manipulations/movements that are used in Swedish massage.

Joint movements (passive and active) active
    resistive/assistive movements
Kneading (petrissage/kneading, fulling, and skin rolling
Effleurage/gliding (deep, superficial, aura stroking)
Touching (superficial and deep)
Friction (vibration, wringing, circular friction, cross-
    fiber/transverse) compression
    rolling, chucking, and wringing
Percussion (tapping, slapping, cupping, hacking and
beating)

520. How are vigorous manipulations applied?

In a quick rhythm

521. Where on the body would you apply light manipulations?

Over the thin tissues i.e. behind knees, around the eyes

522. Where on the body would you apply heavy manipulations?

On the fleshy parts of the body and for the areas that have thick tissues

SOME IMPORTANT
CONTRAINDICATIONS FOR MASSAGE

You should be very careful and take a history of your clients before doing massage therapy.

Here is a list of some of the contraindications for massage therapy.
LC = Locally Contraindicated)

Abortion (no deep abdominal work)

Aneurysm (not even if you suspect a client who fits the profile for aneurysms)

Appendicitis, however after appendicitis operation it can be beneficial with Dr's permission

Acne (LC, you don't want to spread the infection)

Advanced atherosclerosis

Baker's cysts (LC)

Boils (LC)

Bronchitis (LC)

Bunions (LC)

Burns (LC)

Bursitis(LC)

Cancer (should be done only with physicians approval)

Candidiasis (LC)

Cirrhosis (LC in advanced stages)

Crohn's disease: (LC, some massage with physicians supervision)

Cysts (LC)

Dermatitis (LC)

Edema

Embolism

Encephalitis (if in acute stages)

Endometriosis (LC)

Epilepsy (during seizures)

Erysipelas

Fever

Fibroid Tumors

Fractures (LC

Fungal Infections (LC)

Ganglion cysts (LC)

Gastroenteritis (LC)

Gout (LC)

Headache (due to infection but indicated for tension headaches)

Heart Attack

Hematoma (LC)

Hemophilia

hepatitis (for acute hepatitis)

Hernia (LC)

Herpes simplex (LC)

Herpes zoster

Hives (in acute stages)

Inflammation (acute inflammation) but may be okay or subacute situations

Interstitial cystitis (LC)

Jaundice

Kidney stones

Lice and Mites

Enlarged Liver

Lung Cancer

Lupus (when having acute flares and may be beneficial in subacute stages) ask Dr.

Lyme Disease (in the acute stages)

Lymphangitis

Marfan's Syndrome (get physicians clearance before any massage)

Menigitis

Myositis Ossificans (LC)

Neuritis (LC)

Open Wounds/Sores (LC)

Osteoarthritis (LC)

Osteogenesis Imperfecti

Ovarian cysts (LC)

Paget's Disease

Pelvic inflammatory disease

Peripheral neuropathy (LC)

Peritonitis

Psoriasis (LC) in acute stages

Pyelonephritis

Renal Failure

Rheumatoid Arthritis (during acute stages)

Scar Tissue (LC)

Septic Arthritis

Sinusitis (for acute infections)

Spasms (LC) but indicated

Tendinitis (LC) for acute tendinitis

Tenosynovitis (LC) in acute stages, indicated in subacute stage

Thrombophlebitis

Trigeminal Neuralgia (LC) in acute stage

Torticollis (under physicians supervision)

Tuberculosis (when active) with no infection it is okay under supervision of physician

Ulcerative Colitis (LC) for acute stage

Ulcers (LC)

Urinary Tract infection (only massage when in the subacute stage)

Varicose veins (LC) for extreme veins

Warts (LC) remember it is possible to get warts from other people. It's a virus.

Whiplash (in acute stages)   Indicated for subacute stage

When a name appears and has no (Local Contraindication, LC) or anything by that name it is contraindicated (Always check with a physician on any condition in question)

NUTRIENT	DEFICIENCY SYMPTOMS
Vitamin A	Night blindness, itching, dryness of the eyes
Vitamin B-1	Poor muscular and circulatory performance
Vitamin B-2	Cracks at corner of mouth, light sensitivity of eyes
Vitamin B-6	Fatigue, anemia, and hyper irritability
Vitamin B-12	Red and sore tongue, anemia and general fatigue
Vitamin C	Bruise easily, teeth and gum defects, aching joints
Vitamin D	Softening of bones and teeth, bone curvature in children, and calcium and phosphorous won't absorb
Vitamin E	Red blood cell breakdown, poor circulatory and muscular performance
Vitamin H (biotin)	Non specific skin rash
Vitamin K	Blood won't clot

MINERALS

calcium	Heart palpitations, weakening of bones, muscle cramps, and tooth decay
chromium	Poor glucose intolerance
copper	Anemia with fatigue and weakness, bone changes
iodine	Enlarged thyroid gland in neck
iron	Fatigue, brittle finger nails, weakness due to anemia
magnesium	Confusion, nervousness, become angry easily
maganese	Reproductive abnormalities
potassium	Irregular heartbeat, muscular weakness
selenium	Anemia, irregular heartbeat
zinc	Slow to heal wounds, poor appetite, loss of sens of taste

SOME COMMON BUSINESS PRACTICES TO REMEMBER

Keeping accurate records is essential to maintain a successful business. There are several reasons for keeping records. It lets you know what your expenses are, it records the progress of your business. Also your state has certain requirements you must pertaining to taxes, employees, etc.

Your business location is important, be zoned properly, have enough room for you and your client, a clean bathroom, clean shower, fresh linens at all times, and you should have a shower in your bathroom and proper drainage in the shower.

Know the difference between sole proprietorship (a business owned and operated by you alone); a partnership (combines two or more individuals); corporation (managed by several individuals/board of directors) and in a corporation the profits are shared by the stock holders in a corporation. In a sole proprietorship and partnership you are responsible for the liabilities and expenses and all involvements of the business.

You will be required to have permits, business license, massage license, sales tax permit, EIN (employer's identification number) planning and zoning permits, etc. You need to carry insurance in order to protect your business. Some of the insurance you should carry are malpractice liability insurance, liability insurance, automobile insurance, fire/theft insurance, medical/health insurance and worker's comp insurance.

There are several startup costs with any business. You should consider the following costs:
printing and advertising
license and insurance
rent or lease
supplies, furniture, decorating costs
phone bills (business phone)

Remember the three R's
Request = request referrals
Reward= reward the person who sends you a referral
Reciprocate= exchange services from anyone who sends you a referral

Always maintain a pleasant attitude with your clients
Always act in a profession manner
Important: Be sure and check what your state laws are pertaining to operating a business, what the requirements are, etc.

THE IMPORTANCE OF MEDICAL HISTORY FORMS

It is very important for you to have a client fill out a Medical Intake Form. When you go to a physician's office for the first time you are required to fill out a Medical History Form.

It is just as important for you to have a prospective client fill out a form before you determine if they should have a massage.

Did you know there are over 80 contraindications for massage therapy and bodywork? There are many you should be aware of. They are listed in this book. I have provided a sample form for you following this information. There are many reasons for having a prospective client fill out the intake form, and to interview your client to determine their needs, expectations, as well as setting your own policies and boundaries. Some of the reasons are:

- you need to explain the procedures after you have reviewed the intake form
- you need to ask specific/pertinent questions
- you need to listen to your clients responses
- determine the type of treatment
- be professional, courteous as well as sensitive
- be specific about the kind of therapy/treatment
- ask what you client expects from the treatment/s
- be prepared to answer questions about your training, credentials and treatments
  you provide and the expected results
- remember to start all of your sessions with questions to determine any changes that may have occurred since their last treatment
- sexual boundaries should be clearly stated
- professional fees should be stated prior to any treatments
- clearly state what your policy is for canceled and/or late appointments
- you may wish to have on your intake form a disclaimer whereby your services are not to be confused in any way as replacing medical treatment from their physician

The sample intake form follows.

[SAMPLE] MASSAGE THERAPY AND BODYWORK INTAKE FORM

Name_____   Birth Date_____

Address_____   Telephone (   )_____

City/State/Zip_____   Business (   )_____

Occupation_____   Social Security #_____

Male_____ Female_____ . Is Mother living? _____ Is Father living?_____

How did you find out about my service? _____

Was there a specific reason for seeking massage therapy?_____

Have you have massage treatments before?_____ If so, by whom?_____

What is your reason for desiring massage treatments?_____

Were you referred by someone?_____By whom?_____

How would you describe your general health?_____

_____

Are you currently under a health care professional/s? _____ If so, please list them.

Name_____   Name_____

Phone Number_____   Phone Number_____

_____

Are you currently taking any medication? _____If so, list all medications including hormone

replacement therapy, Aspirin, Advil, herbs, and any over the counter pills, etc. _____

_____

May I have permission to contact your health care professional/s, therapist/s for further

evaluation?_____

Have you had any serious operations, traumatic accidents, chronic illness, chronic pain, chronic virus

infections, and have you been under the care of a psychotherapist, psychiatrist, counselor, in the past

twelve months?_____ If so, please be specific._____

_____

_____

Has there been any history of the following in your family?

Heart problems   ☐   If so, who?_____

Diabetes   ☐   If so, who?_____

High blood pressure   ☐   If so, who?_____

Low blood pressure   ☐   If so, who?_____

Arthritis   ☐   If so, who?_____

Depression   ☐   If so, who?_____

Cancer   ☐   If so, who?_____

Have you ever been tested for HIV and if so when? _____

In case of an emergency who would I notify?

Name_____   Phone No/s: (   ) _____

Address_____   Phone No/s: (   ) _____

City/State/Zip_____

Have you had any of the following within the past three to four months? There are contraindications for these maladies. Please place a ✓ by each one that would apply.

LC beside a condition would indicate (Locally contraindicated)

Abortion (no deep abdominal work)

Aneurysm (not even if you suspect a client who fits the profile for aneurysms)

Appendicitis, however after appendicitis operation it can be beneficial with Dr's permission

Acne (LC, you don't want to spread the infection)

Advanced atherosclerosis

Baker's cysts (LC)

Boils (LC)

Bronchitis (LC)

Bunions (LC)

Burns (LC)

Bursitis(LC)

Cancer (should be done only with physicians approval)

Candidiasis (LC)

Cirrhosis (LC in advanced stages)

Crohn's disease: (LC, some massage with physicians supervision)

Cysts (LC)

Dermatitis (LC)

Edema

Embolism

Encephalitis (if in acute stages)

Endometriosis (LC)

Epilepsy (during seizures)

Erysipelas

Fever

Fibroid Tumors

Fractures (LC

Fungal Infections (LC)

Ganglion cysts (LC)

Gastroenteritis (LC)

Gout (LC)

Headache (due to infection but indicated for tension headaches)

Heart Attack

Hematoma (LC)

Hemophilia

hepatitis (for acute hepatitis)

Hernia (LC)

Herpes simplex (LC)

Herpes zoster

Hives (in acute stages)

Inflammation (acute inflammation) but may be okay or subacute situations

Interstitial cystitis (LC)

Jaundice

Kidney stones

Lice and Mites

Enlarged Liver

Lung Cancer

Lupus (when having acute flares and may be beneficial in subacute stages) ask Dr.

Lyme Disease (in the acute stages)

Lymphangitis

Marfan's Syndrome (get physicians clearance before any massage)

Menigitis

Myositis Ossificans (LC)

Neuritis (LC)

Open Wounds/Sores (LC)

Osteoarthritis (LC)

Osteogenesis Imperfecti

Ovarian cysts (LC)

Paget's Disease

Pelvic inflammatory disease

Peripheral neuropathy (LC)

Peritonitis

Psoriasis (LC) in acute stages

Pyelonephritis

Renal Failure

Rheumatoid Arthritis (during acute stages)

Scar Tissue (LC)

Septic Arthritis

Sinusitis (for acute infections)

Spasms (LC) but indicated

Tendinitis (LC) for acute tendinitis

Tenosynovitis (LC) in acute stages, indicated in subacute stage

Thrombophlebitis

Trigeminal Neuralgia (LC) in acute stage

Torticollis (under physicians supervision)

Tuberculosis (when active) with no infection it is okay under supervision of physician

Ulcerative Colitis (LC) for acute stage

Ulcers (LC)

Urinary Tract infection (only massage when in the subacute stage)

Varicose veins (LC) for extreme veins

Warts (LC) remember it is possible to get warts from other people. It's a virus.

Whiplash (in acute stages) Indicated for subacute stage

When a name appears and has no (Local Contraindication, LC) or anything by that name it is contraindicated (Always check with a physician on any condition in question)

_____

I have filled out the Intake Form to be best of my ability and understand that massage therapy treatments are not meant to replace a Doctor's treatment. I also understand that massage and bodywork treatments are considered to be an additional aid in the helping me to improve and/or maintain a healthy body. I have also been told by the therapist that all information discussed during treatments are to remain confidential.   I also understand if I fail to cancel any appointments 24 hours prior to a scheduled appointment, I will be responsible for paying the full fee. If an emergency prevents my calling to cancel I understand I will not be charged.

Signature_____ Date_____

THIS IS JUST A SAMPLE FORM AND YOU MAY WANT TO IMPROVISE

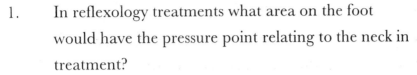

SECTION II
CONTINUATION OF QUESTIONS
ASKED ON PREVIOUS NATIONAL EXAMS

1. In reflexology treatments what area on the foot
    would have the pressure point relating to the neck in
    treatment?
    big toe, base of big toe

2. In massage treatment is it a general practice to
    massage by muscle groups?
    yes

3. Is the back effleuraged before petrissage movement?
    yes

4. Should you always be in a standing position while
    massaging a patient?
    No

5. What is Aroma Therapy?
    **various scents which are added to massage
    lubricants or used in a vapor type of machine which
    has either a stimulating or relaxing effect**

6. What are meridians and how many regular meridians are there?

oriental philosophy/medical science believe that meridians are a system of pathways or channels pertaining to energy (ki) that circulates in a network of channels and collateral in the body. There are 12 regular or main meridians.

7. Name at least 4 benefits of good posture.

improves circulation, appearance, prevents fatigue and backaches, and better on your muscles and joints

8. Where does Yoga originate?
India

9. It is important to exercise when dieting for weight loss, and if so give the reason why?
Yes, because it firms as well as proportions the body as it burns calories

10. What is one of the most popular forms of exercise and list at least 2 benefits?

walking, because there is no equipment required and it improves your circulation and gives you an increase in the intake of oxygen and expels carbon dioxide.

11. What is TMJ dysfunction and how can you treat it?
    TMJ is temporomandibular joint. The mandibular, which plays an important role in jaw pain, has muscles that are attached to the mandibular and if there are spasms in this area the jaw point (in pressure point therapy) can well respond to pressure. Often the diagnosis is followed by grinding down teeth.

12. What is torticollis?
    Latin term for twisted neck. (tortus) twisted (collis) neck

13. What are some of the benefits of lymphatic massage/drainage?
    purifies and regenerates tissues, expedites the balance of the body's internal chemistry, helps to balance the functions of all body organs as well as the immune system.

14.   True or False. Damaged tissue can be carried away during massage, and circulation of blood enables the nutrients to enter the damaged area helping the healing process.
TRUE

15.   What role does the liver, pancreas and glands in the small intestine play in the digestion process?
they supply digestive secretions

16.   Define pathogenic.
It is harmful bacteria

17.   What is the longest muscle in the body, and where is it located?
sartorius -located in the leg (thigh)

18.   Give the definition of a bone.
a bone is a form of dense connective tissue which supports the muscles of the body and protects delicate internal structures, and produces blood cells.

19.   What is Reflexology?
reflexology is the application of applying pressure

to a reflex point (usually on the hands and feet) to relieve tension, improve blood supply to certain regions of the body to help normalize body functions.

20. What do enzymes do?
aid in digestion

21. Name some of the benefits of a facial massage.
helps to keep the muscles toned, increases circulation of blood, and keeps the oil and sweat glands functioning properly

22. Describe what a centripetal movement is.
a centripetal movement is a strong pressure directed towards a center i.e. the heart and it follows the direction of the blood current

23. True or False. Light rays are very beneficial in the treatment of varicose veins.
FALSE

24. Define ligament.
connective tissue connecting bones

25.   True or False. Diastolic is a higher reading than
       systolic.
       FALSE

26.   Name at least 4 ethical codes pertaining to massage
       therapy.
       (1) have a good understand of massage
       (2) keep your appointments
       (3) do not take advantage of a client
       (4) explain the draping to the client before the
       massage.

27.   Name the 3 arches in the foot.
       transverse, medial longitudinal, and lateral

28.   What is a catheter?
       a tube for fluids

29.   What are the 4 basic movements used in massage
       therapy and name the various forms/names of these
       movements?
       (1) percussion =slapping tapping cupping
       hacking beating
       (2) compression = petrissage /friction/
       vibration

(3) joint = passive and active movements

(4) effleurage = stroking with palm of hand or fingertips   Note: Tapotement is also referred to as a tapping movement

30.   Describe what a "passive movement" means in massage.

it is when the joints are massaged and the client does not have to actively move their muscles.

31.   In massage therapy, what is the meaning of "contraindication"?

it would not be advisable to massage because of the client's condition and massage might be harmful more than helpful

32.   Name 3 forms of harmful bacteria.

spirilla, bacilli and cocci

33.   What is Shiatsu?

Shiatsu is a treatment whereby you apply pressure with the ball of your thumb along the meridians to increase circulation.

34.   What is Zygote?

it is fertilized ovum

35. What are the gonads?

sex glands (the ovaries and testes)

36. Name the 3 separate bones of the hip bone.

ilium, ischium, and pubis

37. True or False. The brain is the vital force which controls all the body functions.

TRUE

38. Name the four general classifications of bones and give one example of each.

long = femur, short = patella, irregular = vertebrae, and flat= scapula.

39. True or False. The nerves are the vital force that activates all muscle functions.

TRUE

40. Give the basic principles for draping a client.

any tight clothing should be removed first of all and either a towel or sheet should be used to cover the parts of the body that are not being massaged.

It is important to make sure that the client is not embarrassed or exposed unnecessarily. The purpose is for the client to be comfortable, relaxed and at ease. All of your movements should be very businesslike.

41.   Please be specific in describing how you would drape a female client using the "top cover method".

when the client is on the table have the top cover (can be either and large sheet, or large bath towel), cover the client lengthwise covering the entire body all but the head. When you massage the arm you would fold the top cover exposing only the area that you are massaging. When you massage the leg, you would tuck the cover under the opposite leg positioning the cover tightly (but not too tight) along the inguinal crease

42.   Describe the diaper draping method in detail.

you would use a very large towel (terry towel preferably) for covering the chest and long enough to come to a little bit above the knees of the client. You would ten fold the end of the towel (end just above the knees) into four smooth folds. These folds taper to fit the contours of the body.

The clients leg would then be raised enough to allow the end of the towel to be tucked under the sacrum. The client is then draped properly.

43. Describe in detail how you would drape a female client properly before you would begin an abdominal massage.

    You would fold another towel (in additional to the one covering the body) to cover the breasts and place it over the first towel. Then you would pull the first towel down while you hold the folded towel and place it over the breasts. Then you would take the original first cover of the client and fold the top of this first towel across the client's pelvic area. Then you would raise the client's arm and then tuck the towel (the folded one for the breasts) and tuck this securely under the scapula. Then you would put the client's arm down and follow the same procedure for the other arm, etc.

44. How are cold applications beneficial?

    stimulates the nerves - increases movement of body cells - improves your circulation.

45. Name one benefit of a hot water treatment.
increases circulation of blood to the surface of the skin.

46. Name the organs of the respiratory system.
lungs, bronchial tubes, trachea, nose, and mouth.

47. What is another name for the trachea?
windpipe

48. What is Fascia?
a tough connective tissue that has an elastic component and a matrix that is a gelatinous like substance.

49. What is Myofascial Release?
a hands-on technique that applies prolonged light pressure with specific directions into the fascia system.

50. How many bones are found in the upper leg and give the names of these bones?
One. The Femur

51. Is it really necessary to get a medical record of a client?

Yes

52. In Sports/Athletic massage, what are the major applications?

massage before, during and after an event and also during any rehabilitation

53. What are the connecting links between arteries and veins called?

capillaries

54. Name the five divisions of the spine.

cervical vertebrae, thoracic vertebrae, lumbar vertebrae, sacrum vertebrae, and the coccygeal vertebrae (also called the coccyx)

55. Define what muscle tone is.

when muscle fibers are constantly in a state of slight contraction.

56. What part of the body is the Achilles Tendon located?

just above the heel

57. List at least 3 things a massage therapist should do in order to maintain hygiene and sanitation.

    (1) wash hands before and after each treatment

    (2) keep nails short and trimmed so that you won't scratch a client

    (3) have clean sheets, linens, and towels available for each client, and change linens after each treatment

58. Define tissue.

    a group or collection of cells which act together in the performance of a particular function.

59. Define Anatomy.

    anatomy is the study of the structure of the body.

60. Define Physiology?

    physiology is the study of the functions of the body.

61. Where does the digestion of proteins begin turning into amino acids?

    in the stomach

62. Describe what "active movement" is in massage therapy.

the client participates in the exercises in which the voluntary muscles are contracted.

63.   What is Acupuncture and what is an integral part of this type of treatment?

acupuncture is a treatment where the skin is punctured with needles along certain meridians of the body for therapeutic purposes.

64.   Name at least **14** other body therapies or specialized massage techniques other than Swedish Massage therapy.

Rolfing, Feldenkrais, Myofascial Release, Reiki, Trager, Shiatsu, Deep Tissue Technique (Athletic/Sports), Reflexology, Lymphatic Drainage, Structural Integration, Polarity, Acupressure, Cranial Sacral Therapy, Jin Shin Do.

65.   What is hydrotherapy?

water treatments for the external part of the body

66.   When are salt rubs given?

anytime or following a cabinet bath or hot bath

67.   How high can a temperature be in a steam vapor?

140 degrees Fahrenheit

68. True or False. The skin can safely tolerate 120 degrees Fahrenheit.
   FALSE   110 degrees Fahrenheit

69. Name at least 10 parts of the body involved in the process of digestion.
   teeth, tongue, salivary glands, mouth, stomach, liver, gallbladder, pancreas, small intestine and gastric glands.

70. Name a couple of contraindications in Sports/Athletic massage.
   injury, illness or any abnormal condition

71. Name the various massage movements that have a stimulating effect on the nervous system.
   vibration, friction, and percussive movements

72. What can Structural Integration do?
   it can endeavor to bring the physical composition of the body into alignment and balance around a central axis.

73. Can massage relieve anxiety?
   YES

74. Give the complete procedure for massaging the front of the legs.

After applying oil you apply an effleurage stroke with both of your hands beginning at the ankle. Then you apply effleurage to the lateral side of the client's leg with one hand and with the other hand you apply effleurage to the medial part of the leg. Your hands should massage the entire front of the leg and you can begin applying a deeper pressure and your hand would come up to and over the hip and your hand turns as you come back down to the ankle. You would use a lighter (almost featherlike touch) on the movement back down toward the ankle. You can repeat this procedure several times. The second stroke will be a petrissage. You would begin at the ankle and then move upward along the fleshy parts by the tibia up to the knee. You would then apply digital petrissage to the tendon area around the knee. Then you would do some more effleurage strokes.

Now you would begin to massage the knee and you may or may not desire to bend the client's knee. In some cases client's don't like their knees bent. If you bend the knee however, have the foot flat on the

surface of the table and the foot approximately 16-18 inches from the buttocks. You can either sit on the table so the foot will not slide or you can wrap the foot with a towel to keep their leg from moving during the massaging of the knee. Alternate between applying effleurage and petrissage, and friction from their ankle to their knee. You can apply cross fiber friction in areas that seem to be tense. Then apply effleurage from ankle to knee, then to knee, to hip, to groin, and gluteal crease. Do petrissage to the entire thigh. Then friction to whole leg. Then joint movements. Move knee towards chest to stretch out muscles, range of motion should be paid close attention to. Flex the hip by moving the foot toward the client's head by moving your hand around to hold the ankle at the level of the Achilles tendon. Rotate the bent leg laterally, then when you bring the leg back down toward the table make sure that you support the back of the client's leg in order to prevent hyperextension. You can do these strokes several times. After the leg is back on the table in the prone flat position; then with your lateral hand take the heel in your hand and rotate the foot and leg in the hip socket back and forth (like a metronome).

Take your other hand and place it over the client's instep and apply a slight traction. Then shake the leg up and down keeping the heel on the table. Then you apply effleurage to the entire leg several times and end the leg massage with a few feather touch strokes, and repeat this procedure with the other leg.

75. Name 4 gastrointestinal disorders.

    constipation - ulcers - spastic colon - irritable bowel syndrome

76. What is impetigo?

    a skin infection that could be caused by strep or staph

77. What is reflexology?

    it is the application of applying pressure to a reflex point (usually on the hands, feet) to relieve tension, improve the blood supply to certain regions of the body to help normalize body functions.

78. What is Rolfing and what is one benefit of having Rolfing treatments?

    rolfing is a method of structural integration, and a deep connective tissue massage. One benefit is that it increases suppleness of the muscles.

79. True or False. Nonpathogenic bacteria are also harmful.

FALSE: sometimes they are helpful

80. What function does the diaphragm perform?

aids in the expansion and contraction of the lungs

81. Why should the massage therapist explain the draping technique to their client?

it prevents embarrassment to the client as well as the therapist

82. What part of the body are starches digested into the sugar stage?

the mouth

83. What are some of the things that can be relieved by applying shiatsu?

insomnia, high blood pressure, headaches, nervous tension, sore muscles, constipation.

84. What does Shiatsu mean?

pressure of the finger - broken down it means (finger/shi) (atsu/pressure)

85. In sports/athletic massage what are the goals of the pre-event massage and the goals for the post-event massage?

goal for the pre-vent massage is to increase the flexibility and circulation in the areas of the body that are going to be used; the goal in the post-event massage is to increase the circulation in order to clear out the metabolic wastes, to quite the nervous system and to reduce any muscle spasms and/or tension

86. Describe what a Centrifugal movement is.

a movement away from the center causing a decrease in the flow of blood lessening pressure to the heart

87. In heat and lamp treatments what are the 3 rays used?

ultraviolet, visible light and infrared

88. Name one thing that is very important for the massage therapist to do in order to avoid fatigue and backache during treatment?

pay attention to good posture and make sure that the massage table is at the proper level for the therapists height

89. True or False. One of the benefits of a whirlpool bath is a decrease in blood circulation.
FALSE - there is an increase

90. What is a pore, sometimes referred to as a follicle?
a minute opening of the sweat glands on the surface of the skin

91. What are the 2 types of bone tissue?
spongy (cancellous) compact (dense)

92. True or False. Bones receive nourishment through blood vessels that enter through the periosteum into the interior of the bone.
TRUE

93. True or False. A lesion is a structural change in the tissue and can be caused by either injury or disease.
TRUE

94. Can massage relieve anxiety?
Yes

95. What percentage of an adult's body weight is skeletal muscle?
40%

96. What 3 main techniques are used in acupressure?
pressing the pressure points, touching and rubbing these pressure points

97. Where did acupuncture originate?
China

98. What is the main cause of foot problems today?
wearing shoes that are not fitted properly

99. Sports massage is also referred to what other name?
Athletic Massage

100. Name a massage movement/technique that has a calming effect on the nervous system.
petrissage - light effleurage or a very gentle stroking and light friction

101. What should the temperature be in your massage therapy room?
75 to 80 degrees F.

102. What is lymphangiitis?
blood poisoning or inflammation of the lymphatic vessels

103. Define Pathology.

     the part of medicine that is concerned with the structural and functional changes caused by disease.

104. Name the 3 sections of the spine.

     cervical - thoracic - lumbar

105. Name 3 skeletal dysfunctions.

     lordosis (swayback) - scoliosis (an abnormality of the spine with pain) - kyphosis (humpback).

106. What lubricates the joints?

     synovial fluid

107. What purpose does cartilage and ligaments serve?
     List the purpose of cartilage first.

     cartilage cushions the bones at joints i.e. preventing jarring between bones and gives shape to the external features on the body i.e. your ear and nose. Ligaments help support bones at the joints i.e. the wrist.

108. What is fossa?

     a depression

109. What is sebum?

the oily secretion/substance that comes from the sebaceous gland

110. What is sinus?

a cavity within a bone

111. Name one function of bone marrow.

bone marrow helps in the nutrition of the bone

112. True or False. A very effective way to bring blood to an area is through the application of ice.

TRUE

113. Define a duct.

a canal for fluids

114. What are the appendages of the skin?

nails -hair and also the sweat/oil glands

115. Name a joint that is immovable.

synarthrotia

116. How would you massage over the bones?

you would follow the form of the bones very carefully

117. What muscle opens the eye?
the levator palpebrae superioris muscle

118. What are the 10 most important systems of the body?
nervous - skeletal - respiratory - reproductive - digestive - circulatory - muscular - endocrine - integumentary and excretory system.

119. The urinary system is part of what system?
excretory system

120. The blood vascular and lymph vascular is part of what system?
circulatory system

121. What is a clear, yellow fluid that bathes cells? **lymph**

122. What are the 4 main anatomic parts of the body?
the extremities, truck, spine and head

123. What does integument mean?
skin or covering

124. A patient comes to you and had just sprained their ankle and there is considerable swelling and a lot of pain. What type of treatment would you give? **Massage above and below the area in an attempt to reduce the swelling and help alleviate the pain.**

125. A 65 year old woman has had arthritis of the spine for several years and she stands in a slightly flexed position. When she tries to stand in a normal position there is a lot of pain. What type of treatment would you give? **massage to relieve pain and any spasms and also heat**

126. A court reporter is recovering from surgery for Carpal Tunnel syndrome. Her left hand is very painful. The finger flexors are stiff and she is having a very hard time using her hand. What type of treatment would you give? **exercise to assist her in regaining use of her hand, massage, and heat treatments**

127. What is meant by reflex effects? **is when your hands stimulate the sensory receptors**

of the skin and subcutaneous tissues which causes
reflex effects. Also lymphatic flow is an effect of
deep pressure treatments by stroking or
compression movements.

128   What is meant by venostasis (syn: phlebostasis) and
       list three contraindications when you would not
       massage situations showing venostasis?
       it is a condition that develops due to muscular
       inactivity whereby gravity inhibits the normal
       venous return towards the heart. You would not
       massage if there is a possibility of spreading
       inflammation, possibility of dislodging a
       thrombus, or if there is this type of obstruction that
       the assistance of massage would not improve the
       venous flow.

129   How do muscles maintain a metabolic balance?
       usually through normal activity…when they
       contract they get rid of toxic products

130.   Define edema and 3-4 causes of edema.
       edema is excess interstitial fluid in the tissues. (1)
       increased resistance to outflow at the venous end of

the capillary bed, (2) decreased resistance to flow through the arterioles and capillary sphincters that supply the capillary bed, and (3) increased gravitational forces.

131. Will massage reduce obesity?
NO

132. Can massage take the place of active exercise.
NO

133. What is a hematoma?
a swelling that contains blood

134. How many ribs are there in the body?
24

135. Define condyle.
a rounded knuckle, or articular surface like prominence usually at a point of articulation or at the extremity of a bone

136. What are bursae?
little sacks lined with synovial membrane and lubricated with synovial fluid

137   Name the movements of the diarthric joints.
**gliding, pivoting, saddle, ball and socket,
hinge movements**

138   Internal rotation means to move where?
medially or toward the midline.

139.   External rotation means to move where?
laterally or away from midline

140.   Hyperextension movement means what?
**to increase the angle beyond the anatomical
position**

141   What does flexion mean?
to decrease the angle at a joint

142.   What does extension mean?
to increase the angle at a joint

143.   What does circumduction mean?
**to move the distal end of an extremity in a circle
while the proximal end remains fixed.**

144   What does adduction mean?

to move a part toward the midline.

145.   What does dorsiflexion mean?

to move the foot upward

146.   What does plantar flexion mean?

to move the foot downward (to extend downward)

147.   What does inversion mean?

to turn the plantar surface toward the midline

148.   What does eversion mean?

to turn the plantar surface away from the midline

149.   What does pronation mean?

to move the palm downward

150.   What does protraction mean?

to move a part of the body forward

151.   What does depression (in movement) mean?

to lower a part of the body

152.   What is fibromyalsia?

a disorder - the musculoskeletal function throwing

the neurovascular system "off balance". Many
factors that can precipitate it are personality,
disordered sleep patterns, occupation, hobbies,
posture, whether, etc.

153. What is the difference between asthma and
bronchitis?
**asthma is a panting - paroxysmal dyspnea
accompanied by the adventitious sounds caused by
a spasm of the bronchial tubes or due to swelling of
their mucous membrane. bronchitis is the
inflammation of bronchial mucous membranes**

154. What is the difference between neuralgia and
neuritis?
**neuralgia is acute pain extending along the course
of one or more nerves and neuritis is inflammation
of a nerve/s usually associated with a degenerative
process.**

155. What causes a duodenal ulcer?
action of gastric juices

156. What is colitis/spastic colon?
inflammation of the colon, attacks occur

paroxysmally accompanied by constipation.
Spastic, colicky pain in midabdomen. Tenacious,
gelatinous mucus and shreds of mucous membrane
may be passed.

157. What are some of the things that you want to ask in
your interviewing a new patient?

**did a physician suggest treatments, have you had
any injuries, accidents, etc. and be sure and cover
all things that may be a contraindication to
treatment before you start a massage. Take
temperature before treatment, and ask for a
complete medical history so you will know if there
is high blood pressure, ulcers, etc.**

158. Define what is the origin of a muscle and what is the
insertion of a muscle.

**the more proximal attachment site of a muscle is
referred to as the origin, and the more distal
attachment site of a muscle is called the insertion.**

159. Name two endangerment sites on the body.

the jugular vein and the eyes

160. Why is it important that once you start a treatment
that it not be interrupted?

you do not want to interrupt any flow of rhythm or cause the patient to become disturbed in anyway

161. Name 6 functions of the skin.

protects the body - regulates the temperature - acts as a excretory and secretory organ - oxygen is taken in and carbon dioxide is discharged through the process called respiration - and -absorption

162. How many bones are in the adult human body and be specific i.e. EXAMPLE: lower extremities (62 bones)?

spine = vertebrae 26 bones, head = face (14) cranium (8) ear (6) hyoid bone (1) 26 bones, thorax = ribs and sternum 25 bones, and the upper extremities 64 bones.

163. What 3 things compose the skeletal system?
ligaments -bones - cartilage

164. What is the largest organ of the body?
the skin

165. Name two main layers of the skin.
dermis & epidermis

166. What are the layers of the epidermis and the epidermis of the palms and soles?

the mucosum, granulosum, lucidum, and stratum corneum, and the palms and soles have the following strata: stratum corneum (horny layer), stratum lucidum (clear layer), stratum granulosum (granular layer), stratum spinosum (prickle cell layer), and stratum gasale (basal cell layer): and the other parts of the body, the stratum lucidum may be absent in some cases.

167. What are the 2 major glands in the skin and tell what the function is of these glands?

sebaceous = secrete sebum, and sudoriferous = excretes sweat

168. What is one of the goals in receiving Rolfing treatments?

to reshape the body's physical posture as well as to realign the muscular and connective tissue.

169. Name the inorganic matter found in bones. **calcium carbonate and calcium phosphate**

170.   Name the organic matter found in bones.
       marrow - blood vessels - bone cells

171.   What is periosteum?
       it is the protective covering of the bone

172.   Define joints.
       joints are the connections between the surfaces of bones

173.   How do most massage therapists begin a massage?
       generally with the client in a face up position unless the client prefers the prone position

174.   Name some contraindications in massage.
       abnormal body temperature, osteoporosis, inflammation (in that particular area) infectious disease, varicose veins, phlebitis, aneurosa, high blood pressure, edema, cancer, intoxication, chronic fatigue, psychosis, hernia.

175.   Name the 12 cranial nerves.

Olfactory

hypoglossal

spinal accessory

optic

oculomotor

facial

acoustic/auditory

vagus/pneumogastric

trochlear

trigeminal/trifacial

glossopharyngeal

abducent

176. What is the first thing that you would do if you suspected a heart attack?

place the individual in a comfortable position

177. Would you use cold applications in the treatment of tendonitis?

YES

178. Entrapment of the peroneal nerve can result from an improper massage technique on the: A. forehead, B. upper arm, C. front of thigh D. back of knee

ANSWER: D. back of knee

179. What are the effects of percussion?
    A.   breaks up adhesions and reduces scar tissue
    B.   aids in shedding of dead skin cells and reduces blemishes
    C.   increases range of motion and strengthens muscle
    D.   tones the muscles and stimulates circulation

    ANSWER: D. tones muscles/stimulates circulation

180. Which massage movement is used to break down the adhesions of a well-healed scar?
    friction

181. Which of the following is a bony landmark on the anterior pelvic girdle?
    A. Sacrum, B. Greater trochanter, C. Ischial tuberosity, or D. Pubic symphysis
    ANSWER: D. pubic symphysis

182. Which of the following is a flexor of the hip?
    A. Piriformis
    B. Biceps femoris

C. Iliopsoas

D. Gluteus maximum

ANSWER: C. Iliopsoas

183. Define what a Trager session consists of.

     A gentle rocking and the movement of muscles, limbs, and joints in order to produce sensory experiences of freedom, ease, and lightness. The therapist uses their hands and mind to communicate a positive experience through the patient's tissue to the central nervous system.

184. Define Yin/Yang.

     Yin/Yang is a Buddhist theory that demonstrates the natural process of continuous change where nothing is of itself, but is seen as aspects of the whole or as two opposites, yet is complementary aspects of existence itself.

185. How long should you take a hot bath?

     no longer than 20 minutes maximum

186. The heart, blood vessels including the arteries, veins, and capillaries are the main part of what?

     the blood-vascular system

187. What is the usual order of massage movements and list these in order?

begins with arms (if the client prefers) or back otherwise, then front of legs, chest, neck, abdomen.

188. What is the name of the main artery of the body?

aorta

189. Should a client be advised to drink plenty of water after a massage treatment and if so explain why or why not?

Yes, the system needs to be washed out because you have stimulated the flow of blood and your body needs the water to flush out the toxins.

190. Name the functions of the following in their order: veins, heart, arteries, capillaries.

veins carry impure blood from the capillaries back to the heart; heart function keeps the blood moving through the body; arteries carry purified blood from the heart to the capillaries; and the capillaries bring nourishment to the cells as well as remove waste products.

191. Plasma, red corpuscles, platelets, and white corpuscles are found where?

in the blood

192. What artery supplies blood to the chest, arm, and shoulder?

axillary artery

193. What muscle moves the scalp?

Epicranius

194. What does the masseter muscle do?

raises the lower jaw

195. What is the principal large artery on the right side of the neck?

right carotid artery

196. What is the function of the pulmonary artery?

divides into left and right branches and it takes the blood into the lungs

197. Venous blood is carried through which artery up to the lungs to be oxygenated and purified?

pulmonary artery

198. There are two sets of nerves that regulate the heartbeat. What are they?

    sympathetic and the vagus nerves

199. Define lacteals.

    they carry chyle from the intestine to the thoracic duct

200. What is phlebitis?

    inflammation of a vein accompanied by swelling and pain

201. What is osteoporosis?

    a disease in which there is a decrease in bone density

202. What three groups of muscles make up the hamstrings?

    the posterior thigh (the long head of biceps femoris, semi-membranosus, and semi tendinosus)

203. What are the gluteals?

    the muscles of the buddocks

204. Name at lease 6 lubricants that are used in therapy.

cocoa butter (used on scar tissue), 70% alcohol (good for stump ends), powder, mineral oil/baby oil, lanolin based cold cream, vegetable oil/olive oil (good for baby massage or for anyone that can use the extra nutrients)

205. What type of treatment would you give to someone who has just had a cast removed after having surgery to relieve recurrent shoulder dislocation?
tapotement, effleurage, and petrissage to deltoid and trapezius in an attempt to increase the circulation and relieve spasm.

206. What type of treatment would you give to a patient that has had severe bursitis in the left shoulder for 2 years?
heat, massage, and exercise to the left shoulder

207. For a patient that has severe lower back pain from a herniated disc with severe sciatica associated, and whenever there are any movements from the right leg which stretches the sciatic nerve, it is very painful. What type of treatment would you give?
petrissage to the lower back area

208. Tell what the following muscles do:

(a) serratus anterior

(b) obliquus capitis inferior

(c) rectus abdominis

(d) trapezius

(e) sacrospinalis

(f) obliquus capitis superior

(g) longus colli

(h) quadratus lumborum

(i) latissimus dorsi

(j) sartorius

(k) pectoralis major

(l) pectoralis minor

(m) intercostales externi

(n) levatores costarum

(o) diaphragm

(p) temporalis

(q) recti muscles

(r) sternocleidomastoideus

(s) psoas major

(t) rhomboid

(u) infra-spinatus

(v) supra-spinatus

(w) deltoid

(x) teres minor

(y) teres major

(z) triceps brachialis

Answers to question 208.

(a) raises ribs in breathing

(b) rotates cranium

(c) compresses the abdomen

(d) draws head backward

(e) keeps your spine erect

(f) draws head backward

(g) rotates the spine

(h) bends the truck of body

(i) draws arm backward

(j) rotates thigh outward and leg inward, bends leg/thigh

(k) draws arm forward and downward

(l) depresses point of shoulder

(m) stretches the chest during breathing

(n) raises the ribs during breathing

(o) main muscle of respiration

(p) raises the lower jaw and presses it against the upper jaw

(q) rotates your eyeball

(r) bends your head to one side and forward

(s) bends trunk on thigh or thigh on trunk

(t) draws shoulder blade backward and upward

(u) rotates arm outwardly

(v) helps to raise the arm side ward

(w) extends and bends the arm

(x) rotates humerus outward

(y) assists in drawing humerus downward and backward

(z) extends the forearm

209. What are muscles attached to?

bones, other muscles, cartilage, ligaments, tendons, skin.

210. What is a characteristic of a amphiarthrotic joint?

it has limited motion

211. Define fascia.

connective tissue covering muscles and separating their layers or groups of layers

212. What is the difference between diarthrotic and synarthrotic joints?

synarthrotic joints are immovable and diarthrotic joints are movable.

213. There are two divisions of the autonomic nervous systems, the sympathetic and the parasympathetic. Which of these expands energy?

the sympathetic

214. How many pairs of cranial nerves are there and how many pairs of spinal nerves are there?

12 pairs cranial and 31 pairs spinal

215. The ulnar nerve supplies what two joints?
elbow and shoulder joints

216. The pneumogastric nerve supplies what?
the heart and lungs

217. The greater occipital nerve supplies what?
the back of the neck

218. The intercostal nerve supplies what?
the upper abdomen

219. What does the sacral nerve supply?
the muscles and skin of the lower extremities

220. What nerve supplies the hip and knee joints?
the obturator nerve

221. What are hormones? **the secretions manufactured by the endocrine glands**

222. Where is the pituitary gland located?
just behind the point of the optic nerve crossing in the brain

223. Name the important endocrine glands.
pituitary, adrenal, sex glands, thyroid, pancreas

224. What are the two divisions of the vascular system?
blood vascular system (heart and blood vessels) and the lymph vascular system (lymph glands and lymphatics)

225. Name two diseases of the blood?
hemophilia and anemia

226. The right atrium of the heart receives impure blood from the what?
vena cava

227. Veins of the abdomen, lower extremities and pelvis empty into what vein?
inferior vena cava

228. Which ventricle does the aorta send blood to all parts of the body except the lungs?
the left ventricle

229. What is the name of the large artery on the left side of the neck?
the left carotid artery

230. The left atrium receives purified blood through what vein?

pulmonary vein

231. The veins from the neck, head, thorax and upper extremities empty into what vein?

superior vena cava

232. What does the pulmonary artery do?

it conveys venous blood from the right ventricle to the lungs

233. What is meant by sanitation?

cleanliness

234. How many bones form the wrist and what are their names?

eight bones called carpal

235. In massage of the lower extremities, the manipulations are applied in what sequence?

effleurage, tapotement, friction, and nerve strokes

236. Why is massage of the chest muscles beneficial?

because you are helping the muscles that assist in respiration, and in this way you will be indirectly helping the lungs to perform their function. It also activates muscles that assist the movements of the arm, as well as that of the shoulders.

237. Why should the client's knees be flexed for abdominal massage?
to relax the abdominal muscles

238. What areas of the body have the thickest skin? **the palms of hands and soles of feet**

239. What is a "Charlie Horse" and how can it be avoided in applying massage?
it is a spastic muscle contraction and can be avoided by not hacking across the muscle.

240. How much pressure should be applied in friction of the thigh muscles?
enough pressure to move the underlying muscles

241. How does massage applied to the spinal area improve the bodily functions?
it activates the nerves and brings fresh blood to

stimulate and nourish the nerves, which branching out from this area are the means used by the brain to carry messages throughout the body.

242. When pressure is applied on the seventh cranial nerve what muscles are activated?

the facial muscles

243. What is meant by the therapeutic field in hydrotherapy?

treatment of condition by use of water

244. What is used in a saline bath?

common salt

245. Describe a twisting manipulation that is applied to the muscles?

you place both of your hands next to each other and push the tissue forward with the palm of one hand as the fingers of the other hand pull the tissue back

246. Define the term "remedial exercises".

it is the application of body movements that maintain or restore normal muscle and joint function

247. How can the therapist avoid straining a joint?
by knowing the types of movements that each joint is capable of performing

248 Why should the therapist avoid the "hacking" transversely across the muscles?
it could cause a Charlie Horse

249. Percussion massaged is used more on what parts of the body?
buttocks, thighs, and areas that are heavily muscled

250. Would you use the hacking motion over the tibia?
no

251. Name the two movements that the shoulder cannot perform.
supination and pronation

252. Explain why you would not want to over stimulate a weak muscle during massage.
it could cause muscle strain and could create some toxic poison

253. What is epistaxis?

a nose bleed

254. How do you know if you have used too much oil in a massage treatment?

because your movements will be difficult

255. What is tonic contraction?

sustained partial contraction of some of a skeletal muscle in response to stretch receptors is called a tone, or tonic contraction

256. What is isotonic? What is isometric contraction?

isotonic is having the same tension, tone or pressure. isometric contraction is the contraction of a muscle in which shortening of the muscle is prevented, and tension is developed and does not result in body movement

257. True or False. Claustrophobia is a fear of heights.

no, it is a fear of being confined in a space

258. True or False. Agoraphobia is a dread or fear of crowds of people.

True

259. Give another name for the Lingual Bone.
hyoid bone

260. What is the difference between peritoneum and periosteum?
periosteum is the membrane that covers the bones and peritoneum is a closed sac composed of a thin sheet of elastic and fibrous tissue that lines the abdominal cavity.

261. Give the normal body temperature and normal external skin temperature.
normal body temp. is 98.6 degrees F, and normal external skin temperature is 92 degrees F

262. What is the difference between protoplasm and proprioceptor?
protoplasm is a jelly like substance within the cell and contains fat, carbohydrates, proteins and mineral salts; and proprioceptor is end organ of a sensory nerve fiber located in muscle and joints

263. What can friction produce?
local hyperemia

264. True or False. Flexion and extension can be performed as passive Range of Motion on the humeroulnar joint.
True

265. Where is the olecranon process found?

in the proximal ulna

266. What is a trigger point?

it is a hyper irritable spot that is painful when pressure is applied

267. When you stimulate an active trigger point what can occur? What to latent trigger points do?

Active trigger points refer pain and tenderness to another part of the body while latent trigger points exhibit pain when pressure is applied and don't refer pain.

268. Are neuromuscular lesions always hypersensitive to pressure?

Yes

269. Neuro-physiological therapies utilize methods of assessing tissues and soft tissue manipulative techniques to do what?

To normalize the tissues and reprogram the neurological loop in order to reduce pain and improve function

270. If you client had arm abduction pain what would be affected?
the deltoid and biceps brachii

271. What are the two basic inhibitory reflexes produced during MET (muscle energy technique) manipulations?
Reciprocal inhibition and isometric relaxation

272. True or False. Isotonic contraction occurs with movement.
TRUE

273. What does SMB stand for?
Structural Muscular Balancing

274. Define what the following contractions are: Isometric, concentric, isotonic, eccentric.
**Isometric occurs with no movement
concentric occurs when the muscle lengthens
isotonic occurs with movement
eccentric occurs when the muscle shortens**.

275. What are the three effects of hydrotherapy on the body?
mechanical, thermal and chemical

276. What are the two categories of proprioceptors and where are each located?

Golgi tendon organs and spindle cells. The Golgi tendon organs are located in the tendon near its connection to the muscle and the spindle cells are located mainly in the belly

277. What is a nerve plexus and where is it located?
A nerve plexus is a gathering of nerves and is located outside of the CNS (Central Nervous System.)

278. When you flex the elbow, what becomes the antagonist?
The triceps

279. Define muscle atrophy.
It is a degenerative process due to muscle disease

280. What is nephron?
the functional unit of the kidney

281. What are two responses to pain?
Physical and psychologial

282. Define mechanoreceptors.
Mechanoreceptors are receptors for vibration and for touch.

283. Define organelle.

An organelle is a discrete structure within a cell, having specialized functions, a distinctive chemical composition and identifying molecular structures.

284. What is mitochondria and what do they produce?

Mitochondria are the principle energy source of the cell and contain the cytochrome enzymes for releasing energy and converting it to useful forms for cell operation. They produce adenosine 5'-triphosphate

285. What muscle initiates walking?

Iliopsoas

286. There are many muscle groups. What consists of the erector spinal group?

Longissimus, spinalis, and iliocostalis

287. What muscles are involved in mastication?

Masseter, temporalis, medial pterygoid, lateral pterygoid

288. Name the group of muscles of the shoulder?

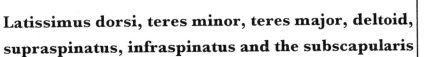

Latissimus dorsi, teres minor, teres major, deltoid, supraspinatus, infraspinatus and the subscapularis

289. What is the most superficial hamstring muscle?
The biceps femoris

290. What is the difference between a sprain and a strain?
A sprain refers to damaged ligaments and a strain refers to damaged muscles and tendons.

291. Name the types of movable joints in the body.
Condyloid or ellipsoid, saddle, gliding, ball and socket, hinge, and pivot joints.

292. Name three immovable joints in the body.
Suture, gomphosis, and synchondrosis

293. What is synarthroses?
It is an immovable cartilaginous joint

294. What does TMJ stand for?
It is a colloquial for temporomandibular joint dysfunction

295. What does TNTC stand for?
Too numerous to count.

296. What is the most superficial quadriceps muscle?
Rectus femoris

297. Name the divisions of the brain, and tell what is the largest portion and the smaller portion of the brain.
Celebrum, cerebellum, and the brain stem. The largest portion is the cerebrum and the smaller portion is the cerebellum.

298. What is inflammation and what are the four principal symptoms and signs of inflammation?
Inflammation is a protective and healing response that happens when tissue has been damaged. The 4 principal systems are heat, pain, redness and swelling.

299. What are the three layers of connective tissue?
Epimysium (covers the muscle), perimysium (separates the muscle bundles, and the endomyseum(surrounds each muscle cell).

300. What is a subluxation?
A incomplete or partial dislocation

301. There are several terms used describing body movement. Define the following:

abduction = movement of a limb or body part further from or away from the midline of the body

adduction = movement of a limb or body part closer to or toward the midline of the body

extension = straightening of a joint or extremity so that the angle between contiguous (adjoning) bones is increased

flexion = bending of a joint or extremity so that the angle between contiguous bones is decreased

eversion = movement of turning a body part outward away from the midline

inversion = movement of turning a body part inward toward the midline

pronation = movement of turning a body to face downward or turning the hand so that the palm is facing downward

supination = movement of turning the body to face upward or turning the hand so that the palm faces upward

302. Name at least 5 positions of the body (positioning terminology).

Anatomic, supine, prone, lateral and oblique

303. What is acetylcholine?

A chemical neurotransmitter found at the myoneural junction.

304. What are the names of the 3 abnormal curves of the spine?

Scoliosis, lordosis and kyphosis

305. Where is red bone marrow found and where is yellow bone marrow found?

Red marrow is found in the ends of the long bones and in flat bones i.e. skull and legs; and yellow marrow is found in he medullary cavity of the long bones.

306. There are two types of bone tissue, cancellous and dense. Where are both of these found?

Dense tissue is found ons the outer portion of the bone just under the periosteum and cancellous tissue is found on the interior of flat bones and in the ends of long bones.

307. What are the three most common types of arthritis?

Rheumatoid, osteoarthritis and gouty arthritis

308. Where is the mitral valve located?

Between the left atrium and left ventricle

QUESTIONS ON
THE CARDIOVASCULAR SYSTEM
AND MISCELLANEOUS QUESTIONS

1. What is carcinoma?

    the most common kind of cancer, arises in the epithelium (the layers of cells covering the body's surface of lining internal organs and various glands

2. What is melanoma?

    an increasingly prevalent form of cancer, starts in the pigment cells located among the epithelial cells of the skin

3. Where does sarcomas originate?

    in the supporting (or connective) tissues of the body, such as bones, muscles and blood vessels

4. Where does leukemia begin?

    in the blood-forming tissues - the bone marrow, lymph nodes and spleen

5. Where are lymphomas born?

    in the cells of the lymph system

CPR Review

1. These common actions can lead to choking.
    a. Drinking alcohol before and during eating
    b. trying to swallow poorly chewed food
    c. walking, playing, running with objects in mouth

2. What is the Heimlich maneuver and please describe it in detail. **It is the abdominal thrust that is used when a person is choking. There is an upward push to the abdomen given to clear the airway of a person with a complete airway obstruction. You ask the person if they are choking and if they can not respond tell them that you are trained in first aid and offer to help. Stand behind the person. The person may be either sitting or standing. Wrap your arms around their waist. Make a fist with one hand. Place the thumb side of your fist against the middle of the person's abdomen, just above the navel and well below the lower tip of the breastbone. Grasp your fist with your other hand. Keeping your elbows out from the person, press your fist into the person's abdomen with a quick upward thrust.**

Be sure that your fist is directly on the middle of the midline of the person's abdomen when you press. Do not direct the thrusts to the right or to the left. Think of each thrust as a separate and distinct attempt to dislodge the object. Repeat the thrusts until the obstruction is cleared or until the person becomes unconscious. I highly suggest you take the American Red Cross Community CPR First Aid Course and review their workbook thoroughly!

3.   What is a heart attack?
It is when one or more of the blood vessels that supply blood to a portion of the heart become blocked. When this happens the blood can't get through to feed that part of the heart. When the flow of oxygen-carrying blood is cut off, the cells of this part of the heart begin to die.

4.   If the heart stops what is this called?
A cardiac arrest.

5.   The first aid for a heart attack is to do what?
recognize the signals of a heart attack, make the person sit or lie down in a comfortable position, and call the EMS system for help.

6. Would you massage a patient with cancer?
    not before consulting with physicians who have knowledge of the case

7. Name the four components of blood.
    red/white blood cells, platelets, and blood plasma

8. How many beats per minute is the (average) heart rate in an adult?
    75 to 80 per minute

9. How many chambers are in the heart.
    four

10. What is another name for "freckles"?
    melanocytes

11. The conductivity of heart tissue is measured by what?
    an electrocardiogram

12. What does the cerebrum preside over?
    will, reasoning, and memory

13. List 16 contraindications.

high blood pressure

low blood pressure

varicose veins

osteoporosis

open sores

diabetes

any break or infection on the skin

cancer

burns

inflammation

fever

asthma

edema (in some cases)

alcohol impairment

extreme frailty

heart disease

LISTED BELOW ARE NAMES THAT YOU SHOULD BECOME FAMILIAR WITH AS EACH ONE IS IMPORTANT IN THE HISTORY OF MASSAGE

Dolores Krieger - developed "The Therapeutic Touch" and (1976, April) Nursing research for a new age. **Nursing Times, 1.**

Jack Meagher - a physical therapist, and pioneer in the field of sports massage (pressure points) and also worked with animals on pressure points

Ruth Rice - a nurse, psychologist, and specialist in early child development developed a specific stroking and massage technique for premature babies.

Iona Marsaa Teeguarden - researcher of acupressure techniques and developed **Jin Shin Do**

Pauline E. Sasaki - teacher of advanced Shiatsu, co-author, translator and known world-wide for her work in Shiatsu

Hippocrates - Father of medicine, the Greek physician

Per Henrik Ling, Swedish massage

Listed below are some additional names that are important and contributed in bodywork in some fashion.

Frances Tappan

Janet Travell

Steven Kitts

Milton Trager

Hwang Ti

Albert Hoffa

Elizabeth Dicke

James B. Mennell

Ambroise Pare

Harving Nissen

Sir William Bennett

Gertrude Beard

Per Henrik Ling

Homer

Siegel and J.M.M. Lucas-Championniere

THESE TERMS RELATE TO PATHOLOGY

Acute "lower back pain"

Adhesions

Atherosclerosis

Arteriosclerosis

AIDS - HIV

Asthma

Migraines

headaches

gastroenteritis

constipation

sinusitis

hernia

PMS - Pre-menstrual syndrome

rotator cuff teat

myocardial infarction

sciatica

kyphosis

plantar fascitis

MS - Multiple Sclerosis

osgood-Schlatters

leukemia

cerebral palsy

parkinson's disease

spinal cord injury - Para, Quad

burns

polymyositis

hypertension

rheumatoid arthritis

cystic fibrosis

systemic lupus erythematosus

congestive heart failure

patellofemoral stress syndrome

hypertrophic scar

ORIGINS, INSERTIONS AND ACTIONS OF MUSCLES
100 Questions and Answers

There are many questions on exams throughout each state in the United States that pertain to the origins, insertions, and actions of muscles. This section will certainly be very beneficial to those of you who are planning on taking any exam, especially the National Exam offered by the AMTA, American Massage Therapy Association.

1. What is the insertion of the zygomaticus major?
    zygomatic bone

2. What is the insertion of the adductor magnus?
    linea aspera

3. What is the insertion of the levator scapula?
    superior angle of scapula

4. What is the insertion of the tibialis anterior?
    first cuneiform and the first metatarsal

5. What is the origin of the temporalis?
    temporal bone

6.   What is the insertion of the trapezius?
      base of spine of scapula, clavicle, and acromion

7.   What is the insertion of the spinalis thoracis?
      spines of middle and upper thoracic vertebrae

8.   What is the insertion of the vastus medialis?
      common tendon of quadriceps femoris also referred to as tibial tuberosity

9.   What is the action of the vastus medialis?
      extends leg and draws patella inward

10.   What is the insertion of the adductor brevis?
      upper third of medial lip of linea aspera of femur (pubis)

11.   What is the insertion of the tensor fascia late?
      iliotibial band of fascia lata

12.   What is the insertion of the extensor digitorum brevis?
      to 1st phalanx of great toe and the tendons of extensor digitorum longus

13.   What is the insertion of the semimembranosus?
posterior medial condyle of the tibia

14.   What is the insertion of the pectineus?
pectineal line of femur

15.   What is the insertion of the soleus?
calcaneus, by way of the Achilles tendon

16.   What is the insertion of the depressor anguli oris?
angle of mouth

17.   What is the insertion of the buccinator? **orbicularis oris**

18.   What is the insertion of the brachialis?
ulnar tuberosity

19.   What is the insertion of the teres minor?
greater tubercle of the humerus

20.   What is the origin of the teres minor?
axillary border of scapula

21.   What is the action of the teres minor?
rotates arm outward

22.   What is the action of the teres major?
rotates arm inward, draws it down and back

23.   What is the insertion of the teres major?
Medial lip of the bicipital groove of the humerus

24.   What is the origin of the teres major?
Inferior angle of the scapula

25.   What is action of the pectoralis major?
flexes, adducts and rotates arm

26.   What is the origin of the pectoralis major?
sternum, clavicle, and cartilages of 1st and 6th ribs.

27.   What is the insertion of the pectoralis major?
great tuberosity of humerus.

28.   What is the insertion of the pectoralis minor?
coracoid process of scapula

29.   What is the insertion of the supraspinatus?
greater tubercle of the humerus

30. What is the action of the infraspinatus?
extension of humerus and lateral rotation

31. What is the insertion of the coracobrachialis?
middle of inner border of humerus

32. What is the origin of the coracobrachialis? **caracoid process of scapula (flexion of shoulder)**

33. What is the insertion of the brachioradialis?
styloid process of radius

34. What is the origin of the brachioradialis?
supracondylar ridge of humerus or sometimes called the shaft of the humerus

35. What is the action of the brachioradialis?
flexes and supinates forearm

36. What is the action of the serratus anterior?
elevates ribs, and rotates scapula

37. What is the origin of the serratus anterior?
upper 8 or 9 ribs

38. What is the insertion of the serratus anterior? **angles and vertebral border of scapula**

39. The triceps brachii is the only posterior upper arm muscle which consists of three heads (long, lateral, and medial). There are 3 origins. Name these origins.
   (1) infraglenoid tubercle of scapula
   (2) humerus below radial groove
   (3) posterior surface of humerus below great tubercle

40. What are the origins of the posterior, middle, and anterior deltoid's and please answer in that order? **spine of scapula, acromion, lateral clavicle**

41. What is the action of the peroneus tertius? **Assists in dorsiflexion and eversion of foot**

42. What is the insertion of the peroneus tertius? **fifth metatarsal bone**

43. What is the origin of the peroneus longus? **upper fibula and external condyle of tibia**

44. What is the insertion of the peroneus brevis? **base of 5th metatarsal bone**

45. What is the origin of the vastus lateralis? **linea aspera to greater trochanter**

46. What is the insertion of the vastus intermedius? **common tendon of quadriceps femoris**

47. What is the insertion of the lumbricales manus? **first phalanx and extensor tendon**

48. What is the action of the abductor pollicis longus? **abducts and assists in extending the thumb**

49. What is the action of the gluteus maximus? **extends and rotates thigh.**

50. What is the origin of the gluteus maximus? **superior curved iliac line and crest, coccyx and sacrum**

51. What is the insertion of the gluteus minimus? **greater trochanter**

52.   What is the action of the gluteus medius?
abducts and rotates the thigh

53.   What is the origin of the gracilis?
symphysis pubis and pubic arch

54.   What is the action of the psoas major?
flexes thigh, adducts and rotates it medially

55.   What is the insertion of the psoas minor?
iliac fascia and iliopectineal tuberosity

56.   What is the origin of the psoas major?
last thoracic and all of the lumbar vertebrae

57.   What is the origin of the vastus lateralis?
linea aspera to greater trochanter

58.   What is the insertion of the vastus lateralis?
common tendon of the quadriceps femoris

59.   What is the action of the vastus lateralis?
extends the knee

60. What is the action of the buccinator?
compresses cheek, and retracts angle of mouth

61. What is the action of the following muscles:
constrictor pharyngis inferior/medius/superior?
narrows the pharynx, as in swallowing

62. What is the origin of the masseter?
zygomatic arch and malar process of superior maxilla

63. What is the action of the mentalis?
elevates and protrudes the lower lip

64. What is the insertion of the mentalis?
integument of chin

65. What is the action of the iliocostalis cervicis?
extends cervical spine

66. What is the origin of the iliocostalis cervicis?
angles of 3rd to 6th ribs

67. What is the action of the iliocostalis lumborum?
extends lumbar spine

68. What is the insertion of the iliocostalis lumborum? **in angles of 5th to 12th ribs**

69. What is the action of interspinales? **supports and extends vertebral column**

70. What is the action of the intertransversarii? **flexes vertebral column**

71. What is the action of the rectus capitis posterior major? **rotates and draws head backward.**

72. What is the origin of the rectus capitis posterior minor? **posterior tubercle of atlas**

73. What is the insertion of the rectus capitis posterior major? **inferior curved line of the occipital bone**

74. What is the action of the rectus capitis posterior minor? **rotates and draws the head backward**

75. What is the action of the cricothyroideus?
tightens the vocal cords

76. What is the action of the obliquus externus abdominis?
contracts abdomen and viscera

77. What is the action of the obliquus internus abdominis?
compresses viscera, flexes the thorax forward

78. What is the action of the quadratus lumborum?
flexes the trunk laterally and forward

79. What is the insertion of the quadratus lumborum?
twelfth rib and the upper lumbar vertebrae

80. What is the origin of the coccygeus?
ischial spine and sacrospinous ligament

81. What is the action of the coccygeus?
supports coccyx, and closes pelvic outlet

82. What is the insertion of the coccygeus?
coccyx and lowest portion of sacrum

83. What is the action of the sphincter ani externus?
closes anus

84. What is the origin of the piriformis?
margins of anterior sacral foramina and great sacrosciatic notch of ilium

85. What is the action of the rectus femoris?
rotates thigh outward

86. What is the origin of the rectus femoris?
Iliac spine, upper margin of acetabulum

87. What is the insertion of the rectus femoris?
base of patella

88. What is the action of the tensor fasciae late?
flexes and rotates the thigh

89. What is the action of the arrectores pilorum?
elevates hairs of the skin "goosebumps"

90. What is the origin of arrectores pilorum?
papillary layer of skin

91. What is the action of the sternocleidomastoid muscles?
rotates and depresses the head

92. What is the action of the platysma?
wrinkles skin of neck and chest, and depresses jaw and lower lip

93. What is the origin of the medial pterygoid?
maxilla

94. What is the action of the hyoglossus?
depresses side of tongue and retracts tongue

95. What is the action of the salpingopharyngeus?
elevates nasopharynx (the soft palate)

96. What is the insertion of the salpingopharyngeus?
the posterior portion of the pharyngopalatinus

97. What is the action of the aryepiglotticus?
closes glottis opening back of tongue

98. What is the insertion of the rhomboids minor?
proximal portion of spine of scapula

99. What is the insertion of the spinalis cervicis?
axis and occasionally the two vertebrae below

100. What does innervation of muscles mean?
the stimulation of a part of the muscle through the action of nerves or the nerve supply of the muscle.

ADDITIONAL QUESTIONS ON HYDROTHERAPY

1.   Define hydrotherapy.

Hydrotherapy is the application of water in any of its three forms (vapor, ice, water) to the body for therapeutic purposes.

2.   What is the purpose of the Russian bath and what are some of the benefits?

The purpose is for causing perspiration as it is a full body steam bath and the benefits are improved metabolism, relaxation and cleansing.

3.   What is the average time or duration for a cold bath, sitz bath/shower?

Approximately three to five minutes

4.   What is cryotherapy?

Application of ice for therapeutic purposes

5.   What are three things cold applications do that are beneficial to the body?

Stimulate nerve, increase activity of body cells, and improve circulation

6. Why would you not endure long periods of cold applications?

    Because they can produce depressing effects

7. What is a contrast bath and what are some of the benefits of a contrast bath?

    A contrast bath is alternating the application of hot and cold baths to a certain part of the body and they help to increase local circulation. The causes an alternating vasoconstriction and vasodilatation of the blood vessels in the area being worked on.

8. Describe was an application of heat would cause and what a local application of heat would cause.

    The application of heat causes an increase in pulse rate, circulation, and white blood cell count. The local application of heat causes relaxation of local musculature and slight analgesia, increased metabolism and leukocyte migration to the area where heat is being applied.

9. What is a slight analgesia?

    It is a neurologic state in which painful stimuli are so moderated that, though still perceived, they are no longer painful.

10. Give two objectives of hydrotherapy baths.

     Stimulation of bodily functions and external cleanliness.

11. What are three benefits of having a cabinet bath treatment?

     Cleansing procedure, induce perspiration and relaxation.

12. Name the three classifications of effects of hydrotherapy on the body.

     Chemical, mechanical and thermal.

13. Give some reasons why the application of ice is beneficial.

     Reduces pain, causes vasoconstriction to limit swelling, acts as an analgesic to reduce pain and is generally beneficial on swollen, inflamed and painful areas.

14. You should NEVER give hot or cold applications when a person has the following:

     **diabetes
     lung disease
     kidney infection
     infectious skin condition
     cardiac impairment
     extremely high or low blood pressure**

15. True or False. Hot water applications improve the condition of the skin by promoting perspiration and by increasing the circulation of the blood to the surface of the skin.

   True

16. What would the temperature of a warm bath be in F and in C degrees, and what would the temperature of a hot bath be in F and in C degrees?

   Warm bath is 95 to 100° F which= 35 to 37.7° C.
   Hot bath is 100° to 115°F, which = 37.7 to 43.3° C

17. What are the three main benefits of a whirlpool bath?

   Soothes the nerves, relaxes the muscles, and increases the blood circulation

18. The skin can safely tolerate _____°F of hot water and approximately _____°F of steam vapor. Water at _____°F over a prolonged period of time would raise the body temperature to a very dangerous level. Fill in the blanks in order.

   115
   140
   110

19.   Define a Swedish Shampoo.

      It is a body bath that cleans the body using either a brush or bath mitten solution of mild soap and warm water and is then followed by rinsing and drying the body.

20.   Is it okay to leave a client alone for long periods of time while they are in a cabinet bath. ?

      NO, you should always be near your client during water treatments.

21.   When is a salt rub usually given?

      After a cabinet bath or after a hot bath. It can even be given as a separate treatment.

22.   Hydrotherapy baths are controlled by three things. What are they?

      Proper temperatures, pressure and duration of the treatments

**LAST MINUTE ADDITIONAL QUESTIONS SENT TO
OUR MEDICAL DIVISION JUST BEFORE THIS BOOK WENT
TO PRESS FOR THE REVISION**
The following questions were given on the Nat'l Exam
May 20th, 2000, and were sent in from 2 states. Some do NOT have
the answers. We wanted you to know what questions are being
included in the exam. GOOD LUCK TO YOU!
Exam. These questions were given in two states in May.

1.   What effect does meditation have on the body?

2.   What effect does yoga have on the body?

3.   Where would you place pillows to support a person lying on the
       massage table on their side? Some of the choices included:
       under their knees and head
       under their head and abdomen
       under their head, abdomen and knees etc.

4.   What acupressure point would you use on the Lung Meridian to
       effect the stomach? Some of the choices were:
       L10, L4, L20

       L4   **This question was somewhat ambigious
                             however the L10 Lung channel relates to the
                             stomach, especially with children who have
                             nutrition problems.**

5.   The heart chakra is:
       (1) Number 5 and blue
       (2) Number 2 and pink
       (3) Number 4 and green - reseach this question

6.   If a person says they have had depression for a long time and
       they think getting this massage will cure them, you should:
       1.   Suggest counseling and do the massage
       2.   refuse the massage
       3.   Agree that it will cure them
       Answer: (a)

7. Why do you elevate a limb during massage?

8. What skin condition might be red and flake off during massage? There were several choices. One was psoriasis which the lady chose. Be sure and research various skin conditions and their appearances, etc.

9. Where does the gall bladder meridian begin? One option in the multiple choice was : outside cover of eye (you must check to see if this is correct) We are just letting you know that this question was on the exam.

10. Where does the spleen meridian begin? One option was large toe. Check this out.

11. What needs to happen to get rid of spasms and cramps in the posterior hamstrings? Precede massage of hamstrings with anterior contraction of the quads.

12. What organ is paired with the stomach meridian? Spleen

13. Which meridian starts in the outside corner of the eye, zigzags and exits at the 4th toe? Gall bladder

14. What do you send a doctor who has referred a patient to you? A progress report.

15. What does HARA mean? A centering place

16. What organ is related to metal? Lung/Large Intestine

17. What meridian is most commonly used for headache relief? L14

18. Which organ meridian is typically used for insomnia and memory? Look this up. Student who sent the questions in was not sure of the answer but it was on the exam.

19. What do you need to do if you are going into business with someone else? Don't tell anyone you are partners. Make sure one of you is spending more money than the other. File a K1 Report to the IRS.

20. In Ayruvedic practices the following is true:
    1. you need to consider the body and mind are separate
    2. the emotions have nothing to do with disease
    answer: the body and mind can not be separated

21. Why does a massage therapist drape a client?
It ensures trust in client and respects client's need for modesty
22. Why is the appearance of a massage therapist important?
Answer: to develop trust and confidence
23. In which layer of skin are the lymph and blood vessels? Dermis
24. What movement helps the functioning of synocial secretion? Friction
25. What part of the body is affected by thoracic outflow syndrome? Arm and neck
26. What does pes anserines mean? Expansions of the sartorius, gracilis, and semi-tendonous insertion at the medial border of the tibial tuberosity
27. What is the function of neurotransmitters? Inhibition
28. Bones touching bones are referred to as what? The student was not sure of the answer however some of the multiple choices were: mushy ends, hard ends, soft ends, lux ends (look this up)
29. What is another name for SOMA? Cell body
30. What systems insure homeostasis?   Respiratory and circulatory   (The choices listed 2 paired systems together for an answer but the student choice the above answer)
31. What does it mean to have NET income? Money minus deductions
32. What oil type is least likely to stain sheets? Water dispersible
33. Therapists avoid injury to themselves by: distributing their weight evenly between forward and back foot.

THIS LAST SECTION QUESTIONS 1-33 WERE INCLUDED AS A LAST MINUTE INSERT. YOU MUST LOOK UP SOME OF THE ANSWERS.   GOOD LUCK ON YOUR EXAM.   OUR COMPANY PAYS STUDENTS FOR QUESTIONS THEY HAD ON THE EXAM THAT WERE NOT IN THIS BOOK.